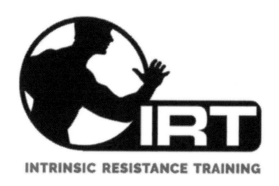

INTRINSIC RESISTANCE TRAINING

HEALTH
&
FITNESS PERSPECTIVE

DISCLAIMER: The reader should consult a physician before starting this or any exercise program. Never work through pain and always listen to your body. If you're in doubt or have any health concerns, get them checked out by a qualified medical professional. Like any activity involving resistance, equipment, balance and environmental factors, working out poses some inherent risk. The authors and publisher advise readers to take full responsibility for their safety and know their limits. Before practicing the skills described in this book, be sure that your equipment is well maintained, and do not take risks beyond your level of experience, aptitude, training, and comfort level.

To my wife, Karoly.

Thank you to all who helped me in this process, especially my family, friends and the clients that inspire me to learn every day.

TABLE OF CONTENTS

Introduction   **1**
    Why "Fitness" As We Know it Isn't Working   9
    Fitness Marketing Madness   13

Intrinsic Resistance Training   17
    How IRT Can Help You   20
    IRT Principles and IN Guidelines   21
    The Basic Plan   22
    Keep Perspective   23

IRT Principle One   24

IRT Principle Two   30

IRT Principle Three   35

IRT Principle Four   46

IRT Principle Five   49

IRT Principle Six   62

IRT Principle Seven   68
    IN Guideline One   69
    IN Guideline Two   71
    IN Guideline Three   72
    IN Guideline Four   74
    IN Guideline Five   75
    IN Guideline Six   76

IRT Practical Application   80
    1. "Quadriplex"   84
    2. "Prone Cobra"   86
    3. "Plank"   88
    4. "Side Plank"   90
    5. "Kneeling Hip Flexor Stretch"   92

Circuit Number One
    1A. "Body Weight Squat"   96
    2A. "Standing Lat Row"   98
    3A. "Standing Chest Press"   100

Circut Number Two
    1B. "Step Up"   102
    2B. "One Arm Lat Row"   104
    3B. "Modified Push Up"   106

Circuit Number Three
    1C. "Hip Hinge"   108
    2C. "Standing high alternating arms Lat Row"   110
    3C. "One Arm Decline Press"   112

Sample Home Workout   114

Circuit Number One
    1A. "Body Weight Squat"   118
    2A. "Band Standing Lat Row"   120
    3A. "Band Split-Stance Chest Press"   122

Circuit Number Two
    1B. "Step Up"   124
    2B. "One Arm Lat Row with Band"   126
    3B. "Modified Push-Up"   128

Circuit Number Three
    1C. "Hip Hinge"   130
    2C. "Standing Lat Row with alternating arms"   132
    3C. "One Arm Chest Press"   134

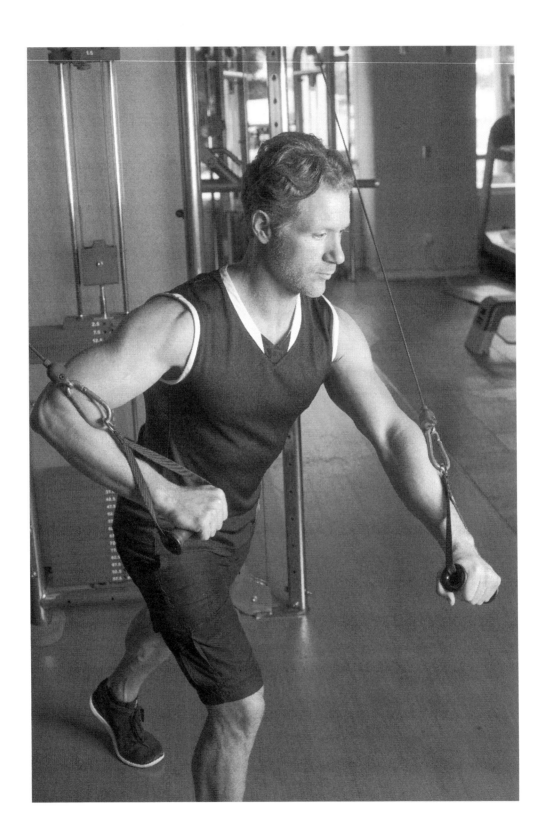

INTRODUCTION

I'm Patrick Spring, the founder of Intrinsic Resistance Training. My mission is to help you practice sound training technique and avoid the mistakes of my early fitness journey, by seeing through the current day fitness facade. This exercise madness has the hardest, newest, sexiest or most unique options fronting as effective training. Personal workout experience and more importantly, years as a top personal trainer, have made it clear that not all forms of exercise are created equal, nor are they beneficial to your overall health and fitness. I've spent over a decade and a half looking for the ideal balance to ensure that working out is helpful rather than harmful to myself and my clients.

When it comes to workouts, more and different is definitely not better and "working through the pain" often ends in disaster. There's no need for another "rah rah captain fitness guy" either, because the fitness industry is overstocked with voices that motivate, without direction or purpose. Intensity is subsequently wasted on the fleeting and futile. What is missing, is a simple and concise practical guide for individuals who want to work hard, but don't want to make their whole life revolve around working out. This book is for those of us who care more about the result than being entertained by the process. Intrinsic Resistance Training (IRT) is founded on a very simple premise: fitness should be supportive to your life, not govern it.

The options of how to work out today are ever expanding. The context of where and when to apply science is supremely important in this information rich world. The principles of IRT will provide you with a broader fitness perspective. This will allow you to assess all your options and free you from relying on the latest workout craze or video to get results. I'm passionate about having you take ownership of your health and fitness, but I understand some people just want to mentally shut down and power through their workout.

However, just like anything else, mindlessly going through the motions won't get you far. Understanding what you're doing and why you're doing it, combined with a consistent, mindful approach is key to long-term success. Unfortunately, there is still confusion when it comes to effective resistance training practice. This book is my contribution to changing that. Let me take you back to two defining moments that formed how I currently view and apply Intrinsic Resistance Training.

My Viking Club High

At sixteen, I was the first and youngest person to get into the Viking Club, the top weight lifting honor at my small high school in the Pacific Northwest. This meant squatting 450 pounds, deadlifting 400 pounds and bench pressing 350 pounds, which had been a serious challenge for my 165-pounds body.

Jogging in the eighties was popular and my dad inspired me to take it up along with body weight exercises as early as nine years of age. I never saw the need for weightlifting until after a broken leg suffered practicing football as a relatively small freshman in high school. Following that, getting bigger and stronger to avoid further injury became a major priority. The day I bench pressed that 350 pounds off my chest, to achieve Viking Club status, was meant to make me invincible. It certainly made all those hours alone in the gym seem totally worth it. Getting that bar stuck on my chest and having to crawl out from under it that one day was just part of my process.

I was convinced wheelbarrow walks of up to 100 yards across the football field which ended with push-ups and eventual face plants were key to this accomplishment. Chin-ups until my hands slipped off the bar and burpees until I could no longer stand, were a badge of honor to me. Of course, it sometimes hurt to walk downhill or sit on a chair after those particularly intense workouts, but that pain was just weakness leaving my body, as far as I was concerned!

I could hardly wait to have my name put up on the Viking Club wall for all to admire. Adding "Mr." to the back of my letterman's jacket was happening for sure now! Social media didn't exist in March of 1990 or I would have posted some adrenaline driven rant to proclaim my new-found place at the top of the fitness food chain, for all posterity. Even if I was feeling a little beat up, it was time to go celebrate in style with my fitness buddies. Carb loading with pizza, pasta and garlic bread at my favorite restaurant was definitely the right decision. One extreme always led to the another in my early fitness endeavors.

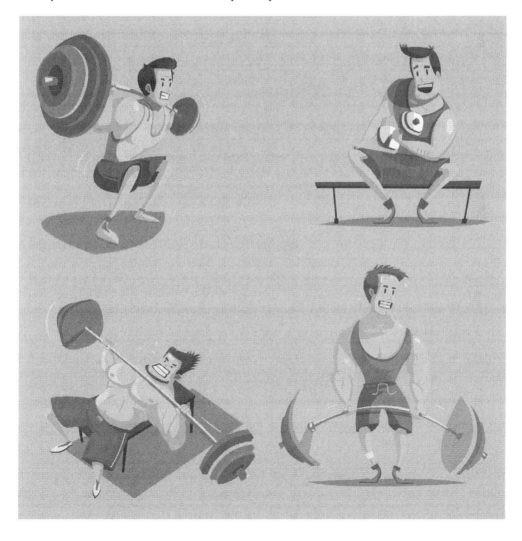

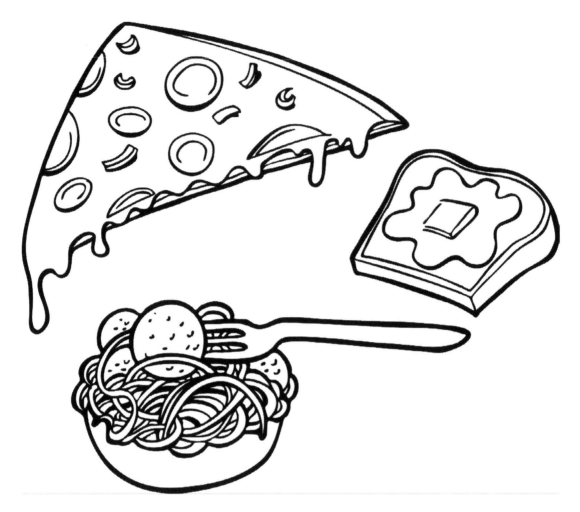

My Garlic Bread Reality Check

Fast forward a decade…. Old habits die hard. When visiting my hometown in the early 2000's, I just had to stop by my favorite pizza place and reconnect with friends for a reunion cheat meal.

For the sake of anonymity, let's refer to my friends as Bevis, Biff and Brian.

Bevis, Biff and I were never late for a meal. We eyed the last piece of garlic bread. I grabbed it before anyone could move.

"Lightning quick reflexes to feed the muscle mass!" I blurted out to mask my embarrassment at eating so much.

"Oh, you're feeding something alright!" Biff replied motioning at my waistline. Bevis started to chuckle.

"Nah, feeding perfection!" I said, laughing at my own defense and adding that it was my awesome long hair that made me look bigger.

"Oh yeah, it's the hair that's bigger alright," they needled me.

"You delicate flowers can watch your figures while I enjoy another grown up portion," I joked, thinking I'd successfully redirected the exchange.

Just then Brian arrived and shouted across the restaurant, "Patrick, looking good!" Brian was the least competitive of our group and never had anything bad to say about anyone. Leave it to him to save the day. He walked over.

"It's been awhile," I acknowledged.

"Yes, you've put on some weight." Brian added in what I could tell he meant as a complementary manner, but also pointing out the obvious that I didn't want to accept. I ignored the satisfied stares and snickers of Bevis and Biff, but started to reflect upon why the jokes had bothered me that night.

After we parted I went back to my parents' house and weighed myself. Sure, this was the first time on a scale in a while, but it was hard to believe that my body weight was actually up fifty pounds. I started to take account of what had led up to this garlic bread incident.

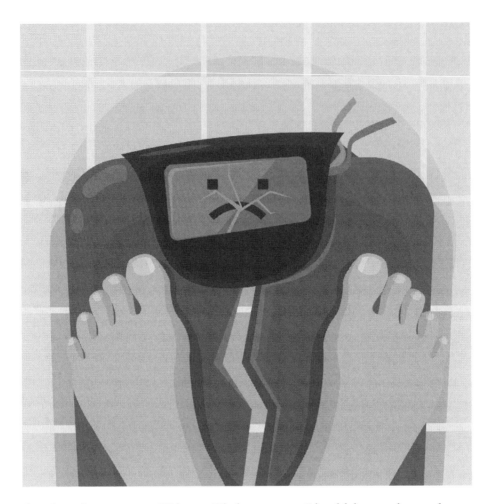

In the decade since my Viking Club victory, I had blown through many workouts and in the process explored numerous forms of fitness. The sheer volume of options kept me entertained, but now exercises that used to feel great, simply hurt. Turning every activity into a fitness challenge was exhausting. I'd been injured often for the sake of doing one too many reps or trying a movement that looked cool, but wasn't natural or healthy for the human body. If I was honest with myself, being kind of a physical wreck became the norm shortly after the Viking Club achievement.

It was ridiculous and frustrating to me that sneezing a few weeks prior had thrown out my upper back. I realized that my desire to try every new style of exercise was actually hurting my overall health and fitness. There were certain things in my routine that had helped me and others that hurt me and I could no longer distinguish between the two. My killer workouts had been put on hold because of injury, but not my cheat meals.

In fact, cheat meals had morphed into cheat days, then full cheat weekends and even cheat weeks. My normal low carb quick fix was becoming less effective and I was simply tired from overtraining.

Had my metabolism slowed down at age twenty-six? Was I going to be one of those guys who always had a bad back? I had ignored my high cholesterol test result as just a fluke the previous month. That night, however, I realized my fitness strategy was no longer working and things were out of control.

At this point you may be asking the question, "How can someone who was born with a "fitness silver spoon" in their mouth and ended up injured with a mouthful of garlic bread, can actually help you?"

I'm grateful for the garlic bread incident, as painful to my ego as it was, because it catapulted me on a path to figure out and resolve my own health and fitness issues.

Although injury was the bane of my existence for many years, it was now more of a blessing than a curse. In the short term, it gave me great motivation to learn more about health and fitness and in the long term, it provided me a refined ability to distinguish effective practice from fitness fluff. Initially, I just wanted the information for myself. Even though I had been a personal trainer in my early twenties and really enjoyed it, I was ready to put that in my past and simply walk the walk.

Since I'd stopped personal training in the mid-nineties, weightlifting had evolved into a whole new beast by the early 2000's. The possibilities seemed endless and the science was suddenly relevant to me. I had to listen to my body even more than someone who had never worked out before or someone who was advanced in years, with the many imbalances that often develop over time. My hard work channeled in the wrong direction had accelerated that process. The wrong exercise, too many repetitions or improper form sent me down a path back to injury.

Somewhere in my personal fitness journey, I lost sight of what should have been natural or "intrinsic" to all movement and exercise. Now I was rediscovering it. I became an expert at properly applying theory into effective practice and paying attention to the context of how and when new modalities should be applied.

The results happened quickly for me and made so much sense, that I was inspired to go back to personal training. Upon re-entering the personal training field, I've earned multiple training and fitness certifications as well as instructed other trainers in the art and science of resistance training. What I've discovered in teaching trainers and training clients is that the enthusiasm one feels early on when inspired by initial progress, makes them more willing and confident to try new things.

The marketing experts know this, capitalize on it and that is part of why most fitness trends that seek to exploit this excitement in the short term, fail the consumer in the long term. A lack of experience also leaves individuals more susceptible to ignoring the bigger health and fitness picture, thus falling for gimmicks based on little if any science.

A vicious cycle ensues leaving customers feeling lost, discouraged and, like a drug, in need of a new fitness fix. I'm particularly sensitive to this nonsense, since personal experience taught me early on that turning ill-suited activities into fitness challenges, is a waste of time and energy. In fact, much of what is currently wrong with the fitness industry mimics my own early missteps.

Why "Fitness" As We Know It Isn't Working:

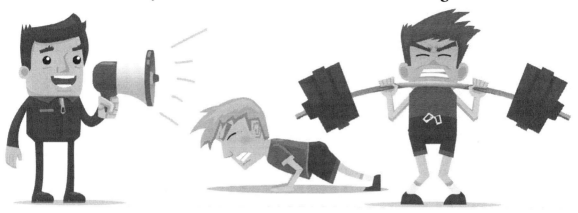

I'm not going to waste time calling out individual companies, but instead I'll point out flawed concepts. This will provide you with more perspective to judge for yourself what strategies follow sound training logic. It is easy to blame a lot of what's wrong with the fitness industry on the popularity of various fitness competitions and their misguided philosophies or lack thereof. Most responsible individuals in the industry agree the concept is problematic at best and extremely dangerous at worst. I do not want to excuse competitive fitness trends, but at least they intentionally or unintentionally spell out that competition or sport is the primary objective. Common sense then tells us that if "winning"/competing with someone else or even yourself is the priority in the workout, it can't also be your health and fitness. In fact, these two goals are often at odds with one another. In short, one must decide if they want to the best at working out or if their workout is to make them better at everything else.

Unfortunately, the blind fervor and ostentatious antics of these cultish fitness contests, make mainstream fitness gurus look relatively reasonable, if not intelligent by comparison. The more subtle and pervasive culprits often get free passes, leaving them completely unaccountable. We need to look at the genesis of another major influence to modern fitness to fully understand how it has been repeatedly misapplied in the wrong context.

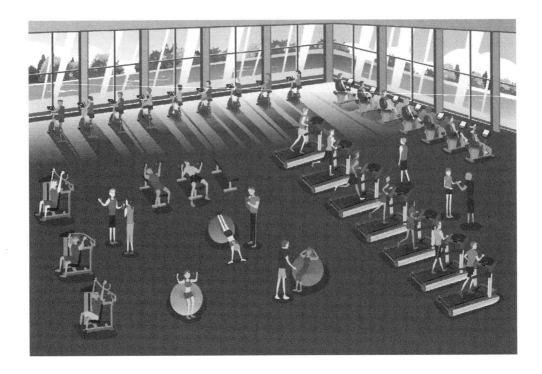

In the late 1990's rehabilitation exercises made their way into mainstream fitness under the name of functional training. They were meant to make daily tasks easier and sometimes, but not always mimicked those daily tasks like sitting down in a chair and standing back up. In some cases, unstable surface training was used for certain populations with body weight to help challenge the "core," usually vaguely meaning abs and lower back. The exercises were specific to the issues of the individual performing them. This application mirrored the research and conditions where these exercises had been shown to be effective.

With time, due to misinterpretation and faulty logic, functional training permeated the whole workout. In the wrong hands, it has become a justification for doing almost any movement in any plane of motion with inappropriate weight and questionable form. The unstable surface training is often thrown into this already volatile mixture for the sake of "core work," to really screw things up. Rope training wearing a weight vest while just barely standing on an exercise ball is an example of mixing ideologies and implementing them in an inappropriate setting. Instead of mere "muscle confusion," general confusion has become the real norm in fitness as individuals add weight to everything from yoga, box jumps, boxing and even spin classes.

Even among educated professionals in the fitness industry there exists contradictions within the context of how and when to apply each modality appropriately. One rehabilitation specialist teaching a class full of personal trainers even argued that one should only train compromised movement patterns and "leave the good ones alone." As a rehabilitation specialist, the logic was sound, but as a trainer loading compromised movement patterns would be disastrous. After fifteen minutes of discussion and a short break, he clarified his stance to make it clear that his comment was not referring to strength training.

Context can account for miscommunication in that instance, but other times presentations are riddled with contradictions that render them simply incoherent. Another instructor spent most of a class debating the minutia of how much weight one should lift to achieve optimal strength. He joked throughout the class that he could lift more than anyone in the room. He also briefly acknowledged that he currently had a weight problem (he used the term "fat") and oh, he just found out he needs shoulder surgery. Wait… What?!

Besides the irony, the takeaway here is to pay less attention to the weight you're using and more attention to what effect each exercise is having on your body. Remember, this guy was teaching a class full of impressionable trainers! Extreme though these examples may be, unfortunately they are all too common.

Taking that into account, it is no surprise that even educated trainers are sometimes perplexed about how to help their clients. They spend hours learning from various rehabilitation specialists how to promote client health and reduce injuries. Then in the main workout, they have their client do too many repetitions of ill-conceived exercises with improper form and too much weight. More specifically a client comes in with limited shoulder mobility and is directed to do a corrective exercise in the warmup to increase shoulder range of motion. Minutes later the same client is out in the middle of the gym struggling to perform a pistol squat on a Bosu ball lifting heavy kettlebells with hunched over posture. Perfect example of a legitimate rehabilitation exercise wasted.

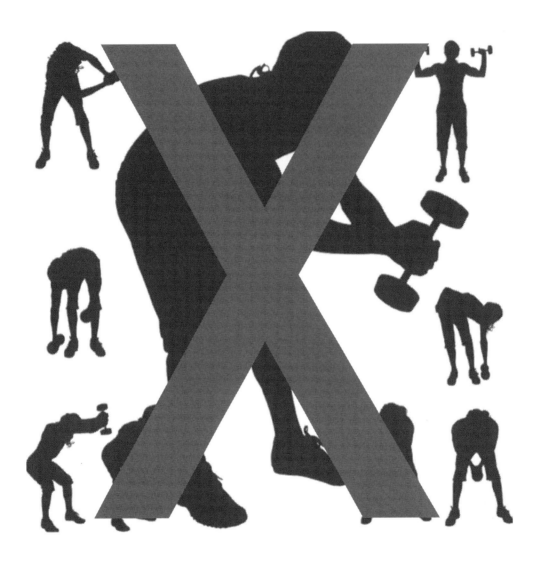

Functional exercises serve only to perpetuate dysfunction when misunderstood and misapplied. Couple their derailed versatility with the high intensity trend in mainstream fitness to rival the fitness competition craze and a dangerous situation arises. Add urgency to help an overweight population with the lucrative nature of this endeavor and it's no wonder that messages can get garbled in translation. Now enter industry marketing to the general population.

Fitness Marketing Madness:

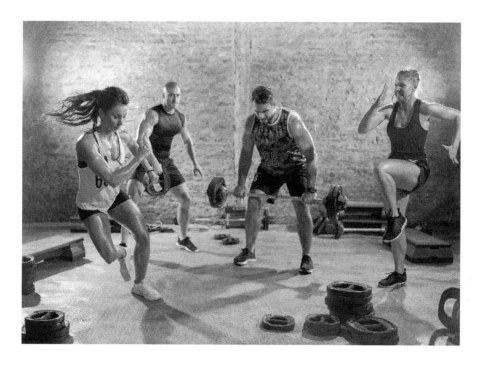

There are many get-fit-quick schemes in the fitness industry that substitute variety for substance and offer convenient timelines. This includes an incoherent mess of celebrity-backed fitness gurus, seasonal trends and fad diets that blur the lines between health and entertainment. Exciting and different is easier to sell than effective and efficient. Big marketing budgets and short-term hype rule the game and overshadow the more sustainable scientific approaches. In this case the confusion is often manufactured and benefits the companies, not the consumer.

I get it! I'm often impressed with how well a fitness commercial is produced, how strong someone is, how lean they look in the after photo or the fitness tricks they perform in the gym or online. The key to my success is that I no longer confuse any of this showmanship with an appropriate workout that's going to help make and keep someone fit for the rest of their lives.

However, when most people look at the latest fitness model, actor or celebrity trainer advertising their flavor of the month fitness routine, they want to believe what they see and hear. Meanwhile the individual in the video has often been training for years, done two a day workouts and avoided carbs for the six weeks prior to this fitness shoot. In some cases, there's even a team of trainers, nutritionist and life coaches to ensure the short-term goal is achieved. Not to mention, the stress of being in a fitness video is enough to make almost anyone "behave perfectly" just until it's over. Try to keep this scenario in mind when you watch fitness programs being advertised online or on television.

Speaking of scenarios, if you're searching for individuals who look fit and can perform amazing physical feats to put in an exercise video, professional athletes are a good place to start. It is no surprise that companies also develop workouts based on how athletes train for their skill set and market it to the general public as an appropriate workout. They don't realize or don't care that genetics and a lifetime of training has led these professionals to where they are physically. In fact, the excessive hours spent on perfecting these unique skill sets are not for the sake of fitness at all. In reality, certain movements may be unnatural or unhealthy especially when you add weight or inappropriate resistance to them. These skill sets are more about technique than a logical way to get in a workout.

Some fitness equipment and programs are inspired by how the military trains. Before you buy into this, think about when the military units use the equipment. Also, realize that the military deliberately pushes their men and women to the extremes. Their lives depend on being able to withstand far more mental and physical pain than any civilian will ever have to endure. You do not need to risk your well-being for the purposes of general health and fitness.

Like professional athletes, these individuals do things for the sake of their profession that are going to break most of our bodies. Also, all too often, it breaks their bodies as well. Boot camps are for eighteen to twenty-year-olds for the most part. Most NFL running backs are done by the time they hit twenty-five. Elite gymnasts hit their peak in their teens and by their mid-twenties they are retired. It's the rare professional basketball player who makes it to forty. Most professional ballet dancers are done at thirty. Most people reading this book want their bodies to serve them for the rest of their lives.

If you play sports for fun, then keep it up, but don't ruin them or your body by trying to make them something they're not. For example, keep playing baseball for fun and improve your skill set to get better, but don't try to turn it into a workout. Practicing fifty swings with a weighted baseball bat on the left and right side is a poor exercise choice. This could be challenging at best and injurious at worst on your off side. It will also definitely slow you down and mess up the timing of your actual swing. That is a lose-lose situation in any book, unless your goal is simply to make money selling entertaining workout ideas.

Some of the same companies offer programs with albeit conflicting ideologies to market to a broader customer base. In these toned-down variations, there still exists an obsession based on flawed logic, which stresses the intensity or difficulty of the process rather than the result it yields. Sadly, the idea that exercise should be painful and produce suffering has become an accepted norm. Haven't you heard people bragging about how sore they are because they got their butt kicked by their trainer or new workout routine? Boasting about how hard or insane the process is with no regard for its effectiveness makes little sense.

I once had a really fit fifty-year-old acquaintance brag to me that he was sore all the time in his shoulders after he did his deep weighted variation of a push-up. He searched for my approval with the rhetorical question, "That at least means you're doing something good, right?"

Upon receiving no affirmation, he walked off proclaiming, "Doing something is better than doing nothing!" This guy's misguided logic ended in neck surgery and he's never looked or felt the same since.

The first lesson is pain is not always indicative of results and the second lesson is doing something rather than nothing is not always good for you, if that something is destroying your body.

Fitness deserves to be held to a higher standard. If someone we knew kept making terrible financial investments and lost all their money, I'm pretty sure we would not agree that, "investing in something is better than nothing, right?"

This preoccupation with the "go hard or go home" approach is distracting, discouraging, and ultimately detracts from long-term health and fitness. I've watched many crazy exercises come and go along with the people who perform them. They usually end in burnout or injury and are often more about showing off and less about the results they yield. Variety should not obscure a lack of substance. Sexy cannot take the place of science. Difficult cannot trump effective. Don't buy into that hype that motivates without purpose or direction.

Working out isn't a contest to see how many reps you can perform or how much weight you can lift. When the workout becomes a competition in and of itself, the equipment, the weight, the reps will always win. There's no prize for overdoing it, especially if the end result is pain, suffering and overeating to mask the misery. This is all a sobering reminder that fitness is a process of following sound principles and always listening to your body. You'll never outrun or "out train" the calories in the long term.

The ideal goal of a workout is this:

You walk out of the gym feeling like you gave your body a challenge, but didn't underdo or overdo it. You feel reset physically, energetic and ready to take on what's next in your day. Think of it as a means to an end. Look at what it's doing for you. Do you feel stronger, more stable and generally healthier after doing it? Is it enabling you to move more freely? Is it making your life easier? This is what an appropriate workout should produce. My clients have come to see that consistent proper movement, with appropriate variation that stimulates the body, yields long-term and sustainable results. That's it.

There is currently a gap between science and accessibility in this industry filled with nonsense. Intrinsic Resistance Training hopes to bridge that gap and help you channel your motivation into something that works long term and will make you want to exercise properly for the rest of your long, strong, healthy life.

Introduction to
Intrinsic Resistance Training

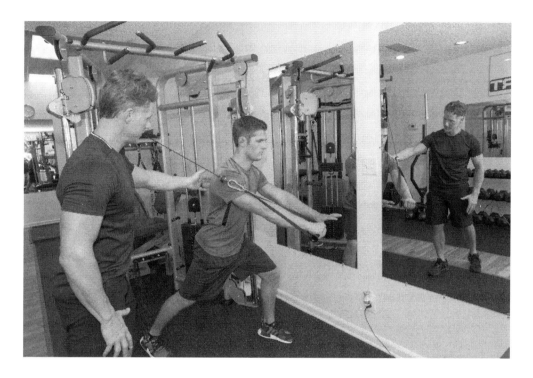

Intrinsic Resistance Training (IRT) is a program for people who want to be as fit as possible for their life OUTSIDE the gym and who are ready to get perspective when it comes to health and fitness. You will be given specific exercises, but more importantly, you will be supplied with the tools to judge for yourself whether any exercise is an essential addition or merely trivial to your progress. IRT distills the scientific basics of resistance training and removes the extraneous. This refined version of resistance training helps you get healthier and stronger, and improve your body composition, cardio, core strength, posture and flexibility all in one workout. The major movement patterns focused on are: *squatting, pulling* and *pushing* exercises, which are the heart and soul of what will transform your body.

IRT provides the principles and the appropriate context of how to load movement in a coherent manner. For example, think of resistance training as akin to lifting something heavy like a large suitcase. You are probably conscious and respectful of its weight. This is the same awareness you should bring to each IRT workout.

In contrast if you're lifting a piece of laundry off the floor, you may be more careless. This is what we want to avoid when loading movements. The more mindful approach will not only help you reduce injury, but it will give you a better and more productive workout. IRT takes what should be innate to all resistance training (but isn't), and reintroduces it. With practice, you become mindful of how appropriate breathing, posture and core engagement are essential parts of every major exercise. This is what constitutes true "core strength." You will master this concept intellectually, but more importantly you will physically know what it feels like as you practice each workout mindfully.

How IRT differs from general resistance training:

Basic resistance training refers to everything from body weight exercises to movements with dumbbells, cables, barbells, machines, kettlebells and many other modalities that provide some form of resistance. General resistance training is a broad enough term to encompass everything from weight machines, Olympic lifting, powerlifting, bodybuilding and loaded functional training. Yes, it even includes mimicking loaded sports skills among the many other poor options mentioned earlier in this book.

In contrast, IRT prioritizes your body's major movement patterns to get results. The focus is on what works best, customized to the health and fitness of the individual, rather than perfecting one kind of lifting. The equipment used will always best suit each exercise or movement pattern.

What further distinguishes IRT from general resistance training, is that other routines focus primarily on what body parts are moving or "working" with little regard for what parts are still and stable. The parts that are still and stable in each exercise like your torso are working too. This concept is essential to proper movement and gives IRT an integrated, holistic approach that is necessary for a healthy body to reach its full potential.

For example, let's say you're going to lift a heavy weight off the ground. Too many people get into trouble by bending down and lifting with their back or letting themselves be pulled into a hunchback position or overarch to compensate for being pulled forward. You might forget to breathe and start letting the weight take over. The weight and gravity will end up directing the movement instead of you controlling it. Trust me, the weight and gravity will not take you to a good and/or healthy position. What you get for all that effort is an inefficient workout at best and a possible injury to boot.

Instead, IRT teaches you to concentrate on maintaining your posture and breathing appropriately. If something is on the ground and you want to pick it up or if you want to lift yourself up off the ground, you're going to do it in a squatting motion. You will bend at your hips, knees and ankles. Your hips will drive or direct the legs. This is usually what is meant by "lifting with your legs and not your back." Not only do I want you stronger, but I want you using appropriate lifting form and avoiding positions where you're vulnerable. As you gain more experience, you will start to recognize and utilize these major movements everywhere when overcoming any form of resistance.

How IRT Can Help You

Since the foundation of IRT is based on how the body should move naturally, its major movement patterns performed with proper breathing, posture and core engagement will create, support and reinforce strength in the human body. When the basics are employed appropriately, they enhance health and fitness, no matter your age or your fitness level. Observe how a variety of clients respond in a similar positive manner to IRT.

Larry: I met him in his late 60's and he wanted to stay healthy, active and get fit. He's currently in his 70's, skis black diamond slopes for fun and runs in half-marathons because he put the right amount of time into the appropriate exercises. IRT prepared him for the activities he loves, including keeping up with his new grandchildren. He no longer stresses about thinking that he has to throw in an extra run or lift heavier weights to burn more calories. His latest undertaking is mini triathlons with his kids who are in their thirties.

Jeffrey: He is in his late 40's. When he first came to see me, he told me that he just wanted to play with his young kids without throwing out his back. He has since lost forty pounds and is now golfing with his teenage daughter and hiking regularly with his younger son. In our last conversation, he had taken up martial arts. He, too, is able to do the things he enjoys and not be tired out from hours of working out with little return. Proper exercise technique has also resulted in no more back pain!

Mimi: She is in her 50's and came to me with a list of all the things she couldn't do, because a lot of things hurt. Certain exercises intimidated her and she wasn't comfortable doing them without a trainer present. She now works out ninety percent of the time independently. By channeling her motivation into the right exercises, she built strength, lost over forty-three pounds, changed her body composition and now feels like she can do almost anything.

Lauren: She is a new mom in her late twenties who was afraid her body would never look the same after her first baby. She was right. One year later, she says that she has never looked or felt this good. Now that she has mastered the principles, she knows exactly what to do in the limited time she has to work out between starting her own business and spending time with her family.

I'm confident that by mastering IRT, you too can have consistent positive results. It will give you tools you can use no matter your age, fitness level or goals for the rest of your life. You will find yourself able to walk into any gym or set up a space at home and know exactly what to do and why. This is important because so many times people go into a gym and have no clue what they are doing and hurt themselves. This is a process to train you in completing these exercises on your own and ultimately being reassured you are doing them properly.

IRT Principles and IN Guidelines

It's now time to get specific and practical. Here's a breakdown of the individual principles of Intrinsic Resistance Training. You'll notice there is also a final principle regarding the importance of nutrition in building and maintaining your healthy body. These principles will inform and maximize every exercise you do.

IRT Principle 1: Listen to Your Body and Work Out Mindfully.

IRT Principle 2: Breathing Acts as your Inner Support for Every Exercise.

IRT Principle 3: Posture is Fundamental to Every Exercise and Maintaining that Posture is What Constitutes True Core Work/ "Core Posture."

IRT Principle 4: Foot Position is Foundational to Every Exercise.

IRT Principle 5: Perform Major Movement Patterns.

IRT Principle 6: Keep It Moving with Cardio and Take Time to Recover.

IRT Principle 7: Proper Nutrition Fuels Results.

After I cover the basic principles, I'll give you a list of different exercises and a sample circuit for home and the gym. You'll see how the movements all fit together and understand the appropriate progression of these movements. You'll also understand how many simple variations you have at your disposal by mixing and matching the major movement patterns (squatting, pulling, and pushing).

That last point is important. The ability to implement basic periodization into your routines, is a technical way of referring to, "mixing up your routine with sets, reps and weight." This approach helps you avoid plateaus, while still providing the consistent foundation you need to reach your goals. It also helps you stay focused by not mindlessly doing the same thing.

The Basic Plan

The workouts are performed in a specific and conscious manner and take about 25-50 minutes depending on your level. As you see, you don't need to practice IRT every day. The following is a sample schedule that provides the potential for maximum results.

Monday: IRT: 25-50 minutes
Tuesday: Cardio: Walk 30-45 minutes
Wednesday: IRT: 25-50minutes
Thursday: Cardio: Walk/Jog 20-30 minutes
Friday: IRT: 25-50minutes
Saturday: Cardio: Walk/Jog/ Sprint 10-15 minutes
Sunday: Recover (you can still be active and enjoy life. Don't feel you need to be a couch potato on this day. With time, you will have more energy and will not want to be totally sedentary.)

Keep Perspective

Spending six out of every seven days on an exercise regime may seem overwhelming at first, but try looking at it from this perspective. There are 10,080 minutes in a week and with this program, you will exercise for approximately 225 minutes. That adds up to slightly more than 2% of your week spent working on your well-being. That doesn't sound like much now, does it? Not to mention that this small amount of time will have a disproportionately beneficial effect on all the other minutes of your week. You will feel and see results which will inspire you to make this a permanent part of your life.

IRT Principle One:

*Learn to Listen to Your Body
and Work Out Mindfully*

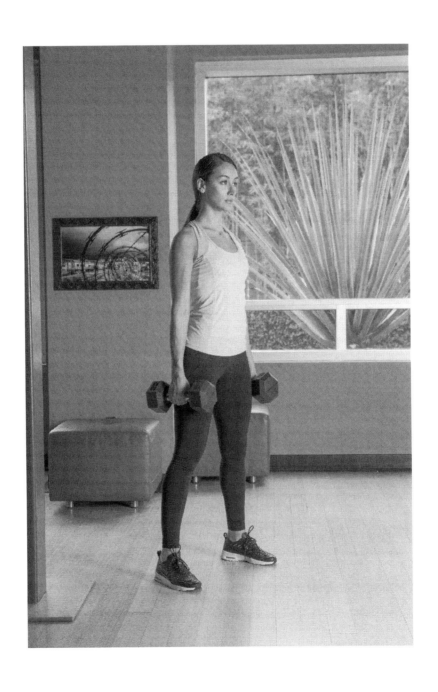

Connecting with your body enables you to get better results and reduces risk of injury. Think of IRT as a map to help you achieve and maintain top health and fitness. It's important when using a map to know where you're at and where you want to go. A map doesn't help if you don't know where you are on it. The same is true in IRT regarding listening to your body. Understanding if you're feeling exercises in the right or wrong areas is essential. Focusing on the right muscle groups can give you better results. You need to know which movements are taking you in the right direction. It's equally important to identify what is counterproductive to your progress. This will take time and practice, but you will get more in tune with your body as you continue to work out mindfully.

> *Listen to your Body General Sidebar*
>
> *Remember that every exercise is ultimately designed to have a beneficial effect on your body, and the quality of the exercise is more important than the quantity. If you feel the exercise in the right areas and can maintain proper form, do as many repetitions as you can. Focusing on the targeted muscle groups will help you get a better workout. However, if you start to feel it in the wrong place and/ or your form breaks down, then stop that exercise and move on. Work out mindfully and don't go through the motions just to "get it done."*

Up until about twenty years ago, we faced one extreme where people would literally do the same exact workout for years, not mixing it up enough, to stimulate the body appropriately. Now we face another extreme, where many people attempt to do a new and different workout every time they exercise. This is a mistake too, because a consistent workout (demand) is necessary to enable the body to adapt.

This is what makes a dancer look different from a football player and jogger different from a sprinter. Changing up the workout too often just for the sake of variety and entertainment, can sabotage your results by not providing a consistent enough stimulus for the body. The goal is to find the happy medium of consistency to promote change and progression to avoid plateauing. Think of it like drinking the appropriate amount water. Too little or too much water can cause major health problems or even death. Just the right amount keeps you feeling your best, neither parched or running to the bathroom every five minutes.

Subtle, coherent changes make all the difference. There are many options to change up your workout but still maintain a consistent demand and force your body to change. This is why IRT works and you don't need to keep adding completely new exercises every week. Varying the weight, sets, reps and tempo are all excellent, efficient ways to periodize and "confuse" your muscles, while still providing your body an ability to adapt with a consistent stimulus. This will become clearer as you review the numerous exercise variations depicted in pictures and video in this book and on the Intrinsic Resistance Training website. www.IRT.Fitness

In the meantime, I'm including periodization or varying your workout within the "Listen to your Body" section. This is because as you add or subtract weight, repetition, sets, and variation to your workout, it becomes even more essential that you be aware of the effects of these changes on your body. When you add weight, you will usually do less repetitions. When you lower weight, you'll usually do more repetitions. When you change up an exercise, you will want to make sure you're still feeling it in the right areas. I've provided specifics below.

Periodization Practical Sidebar

Let me start by defining some basic terms.

Weight - the amount of resistance you use for each exercise
Sets - the number of cycles of repetitions you perform
Reps - the number of individual times you perform an exercise
Tempo - speed of the movement
Bilateral – using both arms or both legs at the same time
Alternating - alternating arms or alternating legs
Unilateral - one arm at a time or one leg at a time

Planes of Motion:
*   Sagittal - in front or in back of your body*
Example: Push-ups or squats
*   Frontal - to the sides of your body*
Example: Lat pulldown or side lunge
*   Transverse - involves a rotational challenge or movements where the hip joint rotates*
Example: One arm rows or transverse step ups

To learn a new exercise, pick a weight that feels relatively easy to perform ten times. Practice doing six repetitions of it with perfect form, feeling the exercise in the targeted muscle group and making each repetition last six seconds. You can break the six seconds into (1 second initial shortening, three second isometric hold and 2 seconds return for tempo/ speed of movement.

The learning phase will be 3 sets of 6 repetitions.
After that simple guidelines to follow are
2-3 sets of 15 repetitions to work on endurance,
3-4 sets of 10 to work on hypertrophy or toning,
4-5 sets of 5 to work on strength

Remember quality always trumps quantity and the repetitions are always guidelines instead of goals. The real goal is to always do just the right amount to make you healthier and stronger.

"The last reps really count!"

I've heard this classic saying misused many times: "those last few reps make the real difference!" This is true, but don't use it as an excuse for terrible form. In fact, it should be the reason to practice your best form, since you want to make sure those last repetitions are counting for the right thing.

Let's say you're working on an exercise that uses the muscles of your upper back. You have proper form and are feeling great. Then you start to tire and the next thing you know, you're feeling excessive tension in your neck and lower back. This is your body's way of telling you to stop. At this point it is counterproductive to do more reps, as you will no longer be working the desired muscle groups, and will be risking injury to other parts of your body.

Simple rule:
When the form breaks down, you're done. If you start feeling it in the wrong muscle group, you're done. Key indicators? Any strain in your lower back, your neck, your knees or your elbow joints. You don't want those areas to be doing the primary work of the exercise.

Don't work through pain

I can't express my feelings more clearly on pain. If you ever feel pain, *STOP!*

It does you no good to work through pain in the wrong areas of the body. If you continually feel pain or are ever unsure about if something is healthy or not, see a qualified medical professional or you could be ignoring or reinforcing a major problem in your body.

Having said that, there is a difference between natural fatigue and burning in the targeted muscle groups that dissipates when you stop exercising and unhealthy shooting, stabbing, throbbing or radiating pain anywhere in the body. You should understand those distinctions clearly to work the right areas in the right way.

Ideally you want to send your brain the message, "Yes, I can do this. This is challenging and I'm ready for the next time." What you don't want to do is work to the point where the message is, "Ouch! All I want to do now is curl up in a little ball on the floor and suck my thumb." Remember, the goal of exercising is to build up strength and stamina for your life outside the gym.

Assess where you're at each moment. This will help you avoid the problems associated with working through pain, or the other extreme of not getting an effective workout, because you gave up too soon. Always listen to your body. It may be elusive at first, but will get easier the more you do it.

IRT Principle Two:

Breath Acts as Your Inner Support in Every Exercise

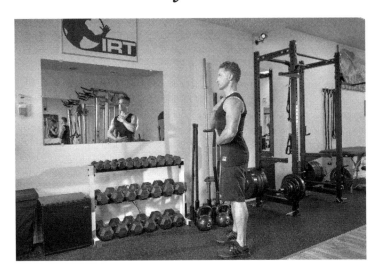

Not only is breathing essential to life, it's the origin of all proper movement. Appropriate breathing is necessary to get in the right state of mind, focused and mindful, instead of the chronic and stressful state of fight or flight. It is also necessary physically to provide you with internal support as you train and move in general.

Having some form of breathing strategy while you exercise may seem like a no-brainer, but you'd be surprised at how many people don't breathe properly. Many people don't even realize that they are holding their breath the whole time they are working out, which detracts from this type of repetitious circuit training. Again, the major movements will be squatting, pulling or pushing exercises and this is a quick reference for how to breathe for each of these respective movements. Principle Five will go into these major movements and why IRT prioritizes them in further detail, but for now just focus on the breathing strategy to match the picture.

Breathing Sidebar

Breathing strategies are often glossed over or completely ignored in mainstream fitness programs. Attention is only paid to it once problems arise, and it then takes much more time and expertise to correct those issues. Do yourself a favor and practice appropriate breathing in every exercise. Proper breathing supports you from within and directly affects your inner core musculature. If you don't breathe correctly, you won't have the internal support to facilitate each movement or exercise.

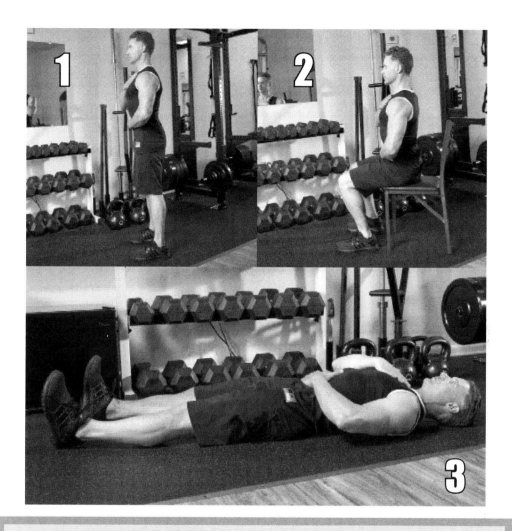

Squat Pattern. Breathe in as you sit down into your squat, stretching your glutes, and breathe out as you stand up shortening your glutes.

Breath in:  Breath out:

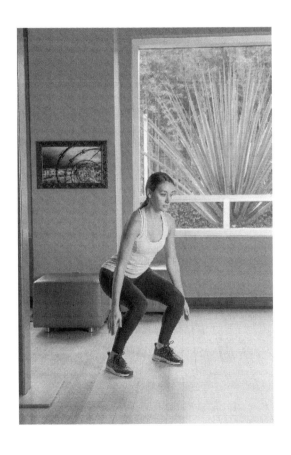 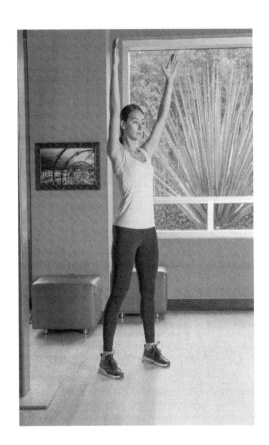

Pull Pattern. Breathe in as you stretch your arms out away from the body and elongate your "lats" and breathe out as you pull the weight back towards your body, shortening your "lat" muscles.

Breath in: Breath out:

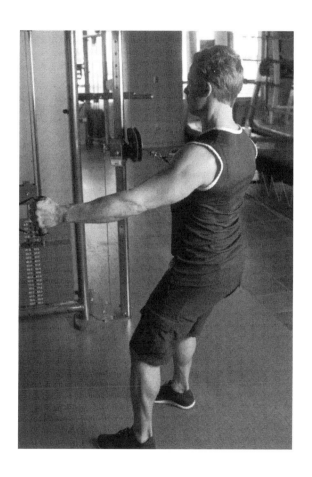
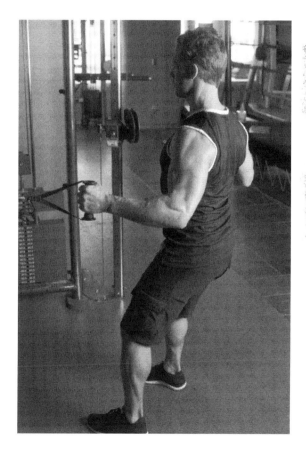

Push Pattern. Breathe in as your arms move back towards your body, stretching your chest muscles, and breathe out as you extend your arms shortening your chest musculature.

Breath in:

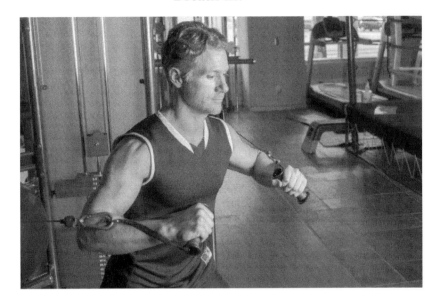

Breath out:

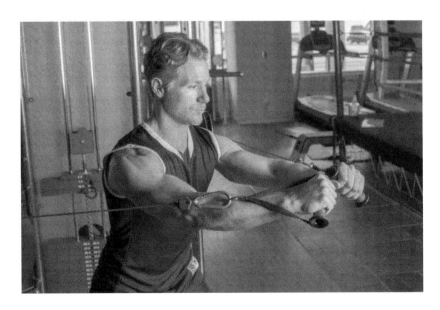

As you can see, you breathe in as the targeted major muscle group is elongated and breathe out as the targeted muscle group is shortened. Again, this is the best strategy for this kind of repetitious exercise.

IRT Principle Three:

Posture is Fundamental to Every Exercise and Maintaining Posture is what Constitutes True Core Work / "Core Posture"

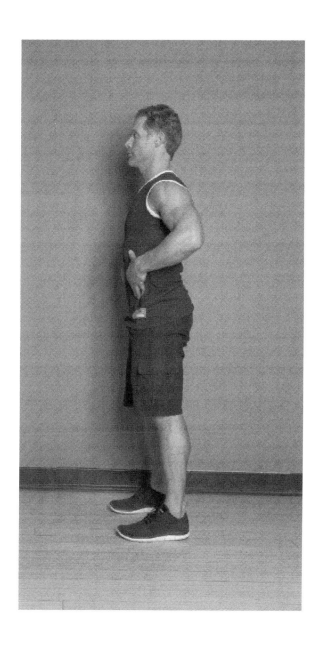

Appropriate alignment of the spine is important in everything we do, be it sitting down, standing up, walking or playing sports. A long, aligned spine is fundamental to loaded movement, because it gives your brain the "all clear" signal, enabling your body to perform at its best. Maintaining proper alignment can also help your muscles work at the right time and in the appropriate capacity. **You will essentially be in neutral alignment from hip to head in all major movements. This means the spinal position will not change or move in segments, but rather remain one stable unit.**

In short, appropriate posture is necessary, because if somebody is out of alignment often enough, no matter how strong, they will ultimately be compromised and suffer diminished performance combined with some form of chronic or acute injury. Although, I'm addressing posture and core separately for the sake of clarifying a couple of helpful exercises, understand in advance that they, along with breathing, are interrelated and need to function together to perform at one's best and reduce the risk of injury.

Posture General Sidebar

One of the best ways to work on alignment and get the right muscles to fire is to think about having a long spine, as if a string coming out from the top of your head is being pulled on. Practice this long spine posture and combine this with your breathing while standing. This will help you become more conscious of what needs to happen in each movement. Below is a diagram of proper posture.

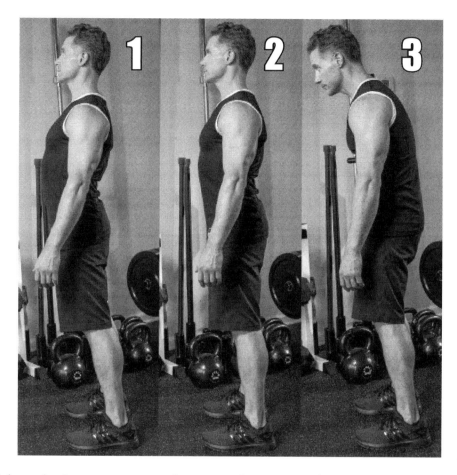

Although there are many elements that can make up or contribute to poor posture, here are some obvious deviations (proper posture demonstrated in Picture 2)

1) **Over-Arching Posture (Sway back)** can be caused by giving into a push pattern or overcompensating in a pull pattern

2) **Proper Posture:** long neck and spine, shoulder blades down, back and around, hips have slight anterior pelvic tilt.

3) **Hunching Posture** can be caused by giving into the pull pattern or overcompensating in push pattern

Below are some extreme though common side leaning compensations, with neutral alignment pictured in the center.

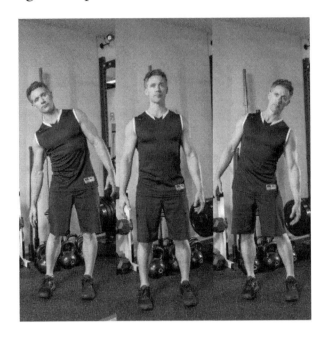

Finally here are some extreme rotational compensations, with neutral alignment pictured in the center.

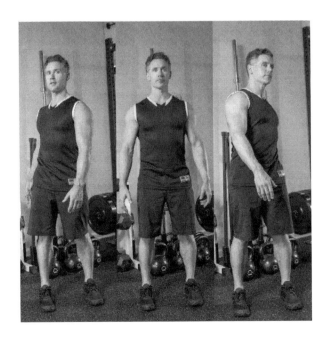

Again, the problematic examples above only represent some obvious general issues. Usually posture is far more complicated and can present itself as combinations of the four compensations above, among many other deviations. These postures will all influence the position of the pelvis (hips for simplicity's sake) and vice versa. I'm not trying to make you an expert in assessing what exactly is going on with your body. Instead the goal is to provide you the perspective to help use the best posture you have, and avoid the obvious deviations.

It is common to see people lifting weights in the gym with no regard for their posture. The focus is often on what's moving, rather than what is still. However, as I mentioned earlier, the parts of the body that are still/stable are just as important as what's moving.

My watchword is this: always stress quality over quantity. If you're doing an exercise with proper posture and start to tire, some natural tendencies are often to hunch over, overarch your back, bend sideways or rotate, strain your neck or do something to shift your body out of alignment. When you start to feel that happening, stop! You're not doing your body or yourself any favors by continuing. Rest, give your body time to recover and then move on. Remember all loaded major movement in IRT is centered around a stable and properly aligned spinal position.

Core is working in every exercise and is referred to as "Core Posture"

My goal in this section is to re-define how most people currently view the "core", one of the most overused and misunderstood words in the fitness world. Many people think of core as a separate part of your body to throw in by "focusing on 10-15 minutes of core" at the end of the workout.

However, the reality is that you're not just working core when you do planks, march, stand on unstable surfaces or do old-school sit-ups. The idea is to be working core in every movement to the degree it is needed. Yes, even and especially when you're squatting. It is literally at the center of all movements. In fact, every exercise when done properly, strengthens your core and reinforces alignment.

When I refer to core, I mean the ability to maintain/stabilize that ideal posture discussed above, aligned from hips through head as one unit in every exercise. **Breathing appropriately and maintaining posture by bracing yourself in opposition to external forces like gravity and resistance of any kind, is what constitutes "core work" or Core Posture.**

This important relationship between breath (for inner support), posture and outer core support is critical to a strong and healthy body. Improving one element will feed into improving all three, because they are all interdependent and rely on one another to function optimally. Each one complements and reinforces the others. Better posture means that the outer core muscles are better aligned to do their job and can also help create ideal conditions for breathing.

Core Posture General Sidebar

In each exercise, stopping yourself (or bracing yourself) from being pulled out of proper alignment and breathing appropriately constitutes core work and is referred to as Core Posture in IRT. Strong Core Posture will allow for greater ability of your arms and legs to produce force when you are squatting, pulling and pushing. Specifically, when you're being pulled backwards, forwards, sideways or into rotation, your Core Posture is challenged in different capacities. Each exercise in IRT is working major muscle groups along with Core Posture.

Core Posture Practical Sidebar

Remember, we do not need maximum core contraction at all times. You do not need to "squeeze" or over-tighten anything. Instead, we want the right amount of core activation at the right time and in the right capacity. Think about having a long spine, and being stable from hip through head in every exercise. When performing major movements, core posture can be broken down into four main challenges that you must overcome to strengthen your core. Please see picures 1-4 on the following pages.

1) Anti-extension (Don't over-arch) illustrated below with extension (arching) challenges.

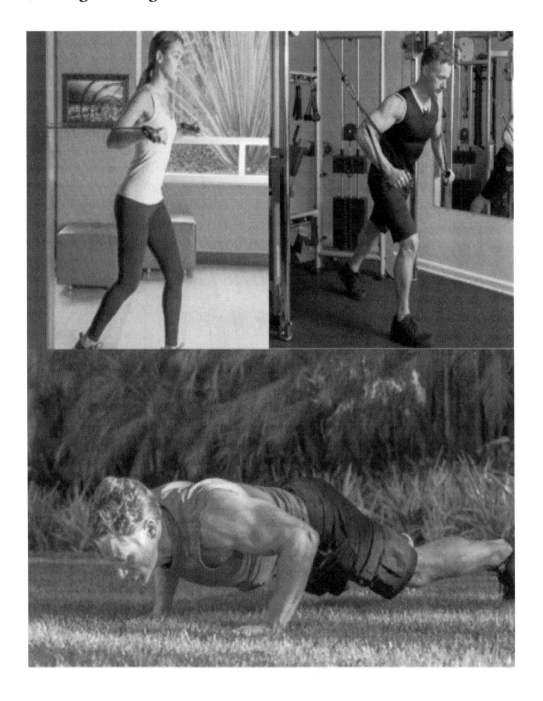

2) Anti-flexion (Don't hunch) illustrated below with flexion (hunching) challenges.

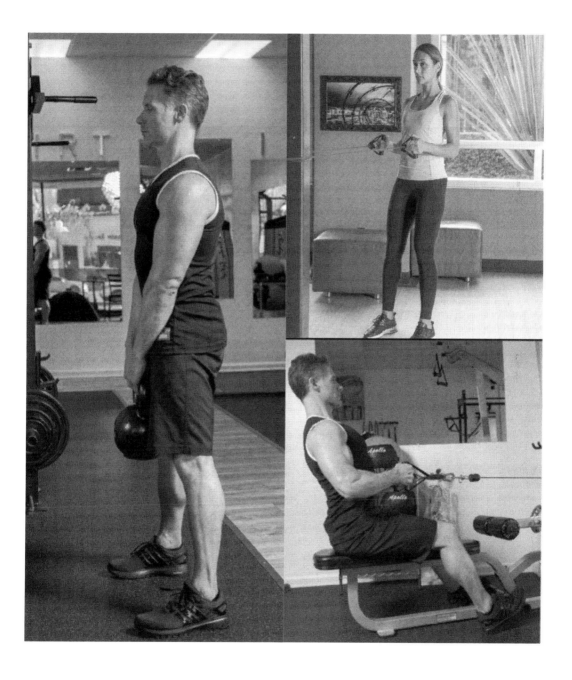

3) Anti-rotation (Don't twist) illustrated below with rotational (twisting) challenges.

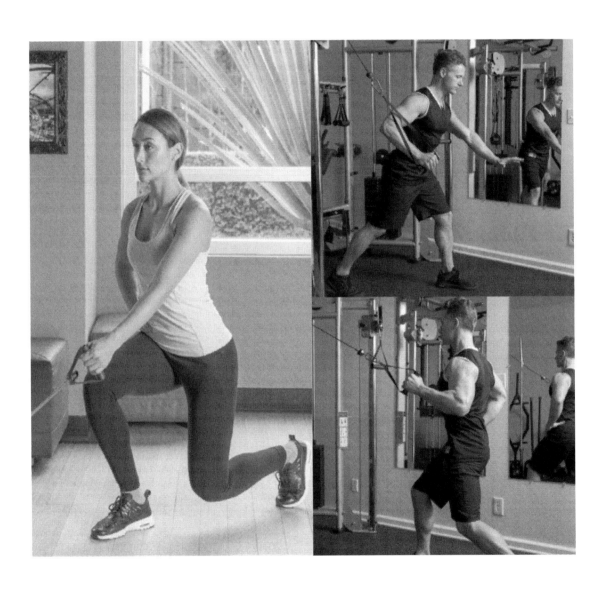

4) Anti-lateral flexion (Don't lean sideways) illustrated below with lateral flexion (side bending) challenges.

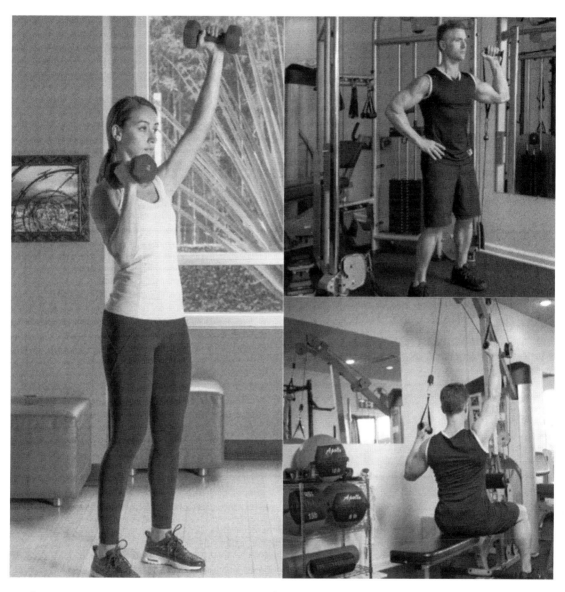

As you can see, *Core Posture* is simply maintaining ideal posture in any number of challenging situations. It is about keeping your spine neutral rather than letting it flex forward, backwards, sideways or twist. Breathing, posture and related core activation all rely on one another to function properly. ***In short, the first two principles breathing and maintaining posture form the foundation of all movement in IRT and are essentially combined into one principle, Core Posture.***

IRT Principle Four:
Stable Foot Position

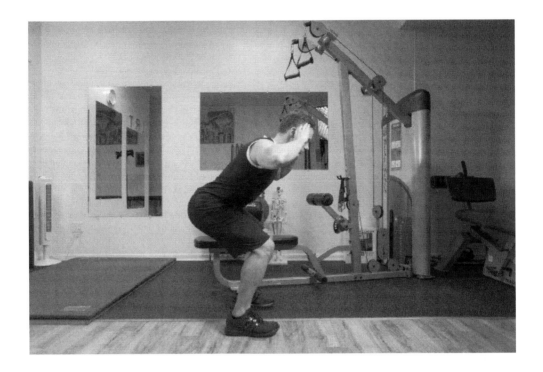

Foot position is literally the foundation to all your **standing** exercises. However, it also profoundly influences laying and sitting positions, so be aware of it in every exercise even if you aren't necessarily standing. **Stable Foot Position** refers to keeping your weight on the three optimal points of contact of the loaded foot/feet. This means standing on your heel, ball of big toe (1st MTP joint), and ball of little toe (5th MTP joint). Make sure that your foot/ground connection remains constant and doesn't roll or collapse in any direction. This concept is always applicable to the loaded leg when standing.

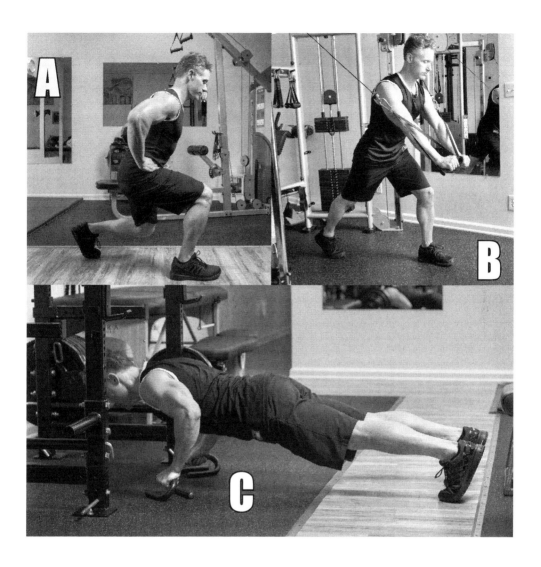

In this traveling lunge example above in photograph A, we are referring to the front leg's foot, which should be placed squarely on the ground. When the emphasis is upper body as in decline cable chest press pictured in photograph B, sometimes the weight will be on the ball of the back foot, to get your body weight behind the exercise.

This is also true for push-ups when your goal is to place most of your body weight on the upper body pictured in photograph C.

If you always strive to stay aware of the bigger picture, these exceptions will make more sense as you proceed.

The feet and their solid placement on the ground are foundational to stability and strength. Having your weight evenly distributed on the heel, the big toe joint and little toe joint is ideal and will result in better hip and spinal alignment. Don't let your feet collapse in or fall outward. Keep the feet active, but not tense.

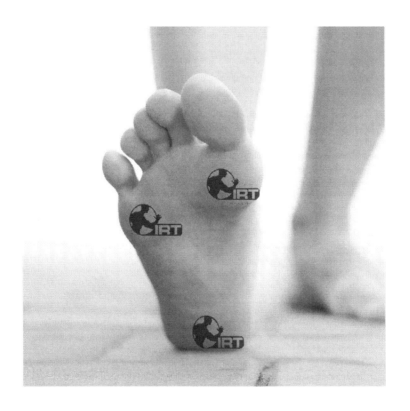

IRT Principle Five:
Perform Major Movement Patterns

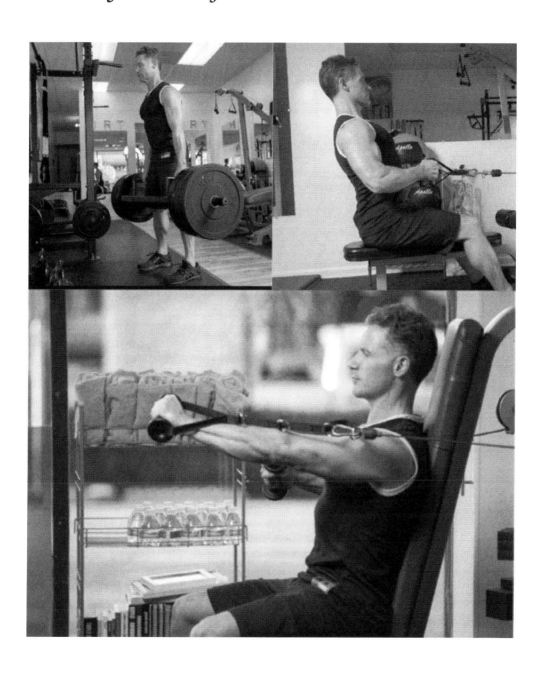

Want results? Make major movement patterns the focus of your workout. Squatting, pulling and pushing movements are where your body is in the most advantageous positions to move any form of resistance including your own body weight. They challenge your body in the capacity that is appropriate for each area, while loaded with resistance. These movement patterns are also more forgiving than exercises that seek to be too specific in targeting smaller muscle groups. The more specific you get with exercise choices, the greater the need generally is to know precisely what is going on with your body and exactly what you are doing. In this forum, the broader approach is safer and more effective.

The order of squat, pull and then push when performing circuits of the three major exercises works best. It allows you to start from the ground up, focusing on the foundation of the body first with squatting. It then enables you to pull thereby warming up shoulders and become more conscious of optimal posture. This will set you up well for your final pushing exercise. The order also avoids leaving you with an overly fatigued torso, upper back and arms as you return to your squatting pattern, after your push pattern. For all of these reasons, the order of squat, pull and push is preferred in IRT.

With each exercise, you reinforce stability in the torso (Core Posture) and mobility in your legs and arms, driven by the major muscle groups (glutes/butt, lats/upper back, pecs/chest). Stability and mobility in the right parts of your body are essential to proper movement and mutually enhance one another. This concept is especially important when adding resistance (dumbbells, cables, kettle bells, etc.) to any exercise.

All major loaded movements will be performed on a stable surface when working to increase your strength. You should keep in mind that if you want to perform at your best, you need a certain amount of stability to do so. Imagine trying to lift a heavy person off the ground. Now imagine trying to do the same on a sheet of ice. If you didn't consciously take it easy and use less force under these circumstances, your body would adjust for you as a protective mechanism. Your ability to lift heavy weight would diminish as it does whenever unstable surfaces are used to train.

Be careful if you decide to use these modalities of when and how you employ them. It's also important to consider this logic when working one leg or arm at a time. The more unstable you get, the less weight you should use. You will employ these options with a lighter weight to challenge the body, but it's important to remember that you never want to feel unstable or awkward in IRT. If it happens, it's the wrong exercise for that day or until you feel comfortable or stable performing it.

Major Movement Patterns General Sidebar

Major movement patterns are basic movements where the body is in an advantageous and safe position to lift weight or maneuver itself around. These major movement patterns all happen to be "compound movements" and they work the biggest muscle groups in your body (glutes, back, chest) and increase muscle building and calorie-burning potential. Compound movements are those that involve multiple joints at a time to perform a task, compared to single-joint movements where one joint is involved at a time. Every major circuit you perform in IRT will be primarily composed of a squatting movement, a pulling movement and a pushing movement, in that order.

Squat, Pull and Push Dynamic Practical Sidebar

Let's get specific about what each exercise works.

Squatting: Works your glutes (butt) and legs. Spine is stable (Core Posture) as you hinge (have mobility) at your hip joint, knee joint and ankle joint.

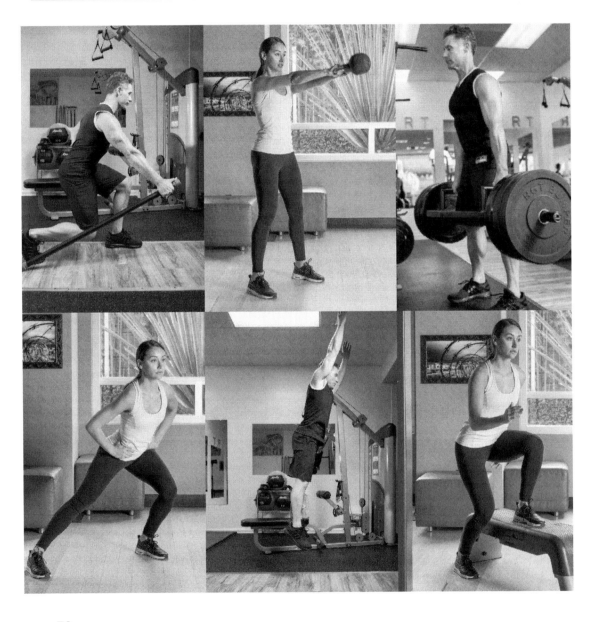

Pulling: Works your upper back muscles (lats) and arms. Spine is stable (Core Posture) as you hinge (have mobility) at your shoulder and elbow joints.

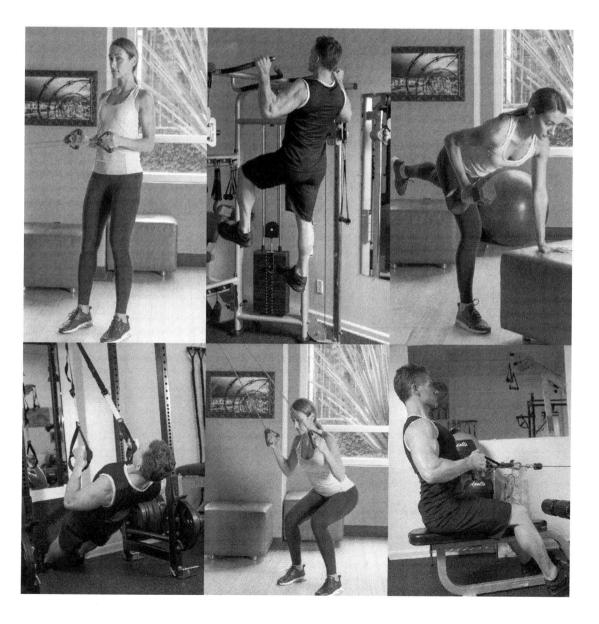

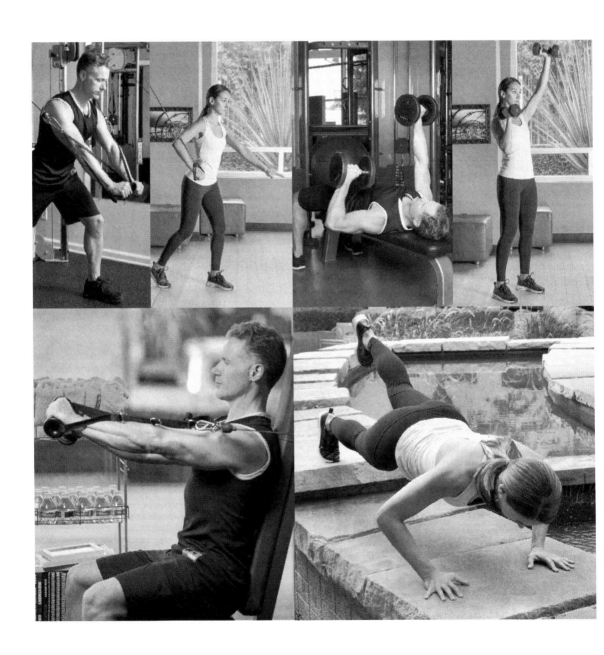

Squat, Pull and Push Practical Preparation

To learn a new exercise, pick a weight that feels relatively easy to perform ten times. For squatting movements, body weight is initially the preference. Practice doing three to six repetitions of it with perfect form, feeling the exercise in the targeted muscle group and making each repetition last six seconds. You can break the six seconds into (one-second initial shortening (concentric), three-second sustained hold (isometric) and two-second return (eccentric) for tempo/ speed of movement.

If you felt the exercises in the corresponding targeted muscle groups, now try holding the exercise for six to ten seconds at a time in the shortened position. Keep paying attention to posture and breathing. Again, this kind of sustained hold is called an isometric exercise and can be done at any time to help you reconnect with proper posture and the targeted muscle group. Isometrics are a great way to get the brain and muscles to communicate more effectively. If you start to feel the exercise in the wrong area or you start to cramp, STOP. Give yourself some time to recover by moving to the next exercise in the circuit and come back to it later.

After you can hold isometrics comfortably for 20 to 30 seconds, the guidelines to follow from the "Listen to your Body" section are reiterated below:
2-3 sets of 15 repetitions to work on endurance,
3-4 sets of 10 to work on hypertrophy it toning,
4-5 sets of 5 to work on strength

At this point, you might still be asking yourself, "What about the rest of my body? I want flat abs and tight triceps. How do I get those with these exercises?"

These are great questions. The answers are deceptively simple. This is why IRT is efficient and effective. Not only are you working major muscle groups when performing these movements, remember you are working your Core Posture as a part of every exercise. That means there is no need to do extra "core work." Not to mention that you are also working other secondary muscle groups as well. Your legs work in every squatting exercise and your arms work in the pulling and pushing patterns. In summation, you're working your entire body in the right capacity at the right time with the three major movement patterns.

Your body takes priority over the equipment you use

One way to ensure that you work things in the right capacity is to utilize the appropriate equipment for the job. IRT allows your body to move freely from stable aligned Core Posture, using equipment that supports natural movement patterns. For example, you will use dumb-bells instead of barbells for certain exercises. A specific example of this is using dumbbells, kettlebells or cables for shoulder press instead of a traditional barbell, because the former allows you move the weight through the optimal range of motion without having to move your head. With a traditional bar on the other hand, you need to move your head forward or backward out of alignment or stop the movement short altogether to avoid hitting yourself in the head with the bar. In other words, if you must alter the exercise to avoid hitting yourself with the equipment, then your focus is on the wrong thing. There is a more efficient option that will facilitate your body's natural movement pattern instead of accommodating the equipment. Here are three quick examples.

As you can see with the barbell, you must either move your head backwards (photograph A) or forward (photograph B) to avoid the bar or stop in a less than optimal range of motion because the bar makes contact with your head when it's in a neutral position (photograph C)

Barbell Shoulder Press
Not Preferred

Dumbbell Shoulder Press
Preferred Method

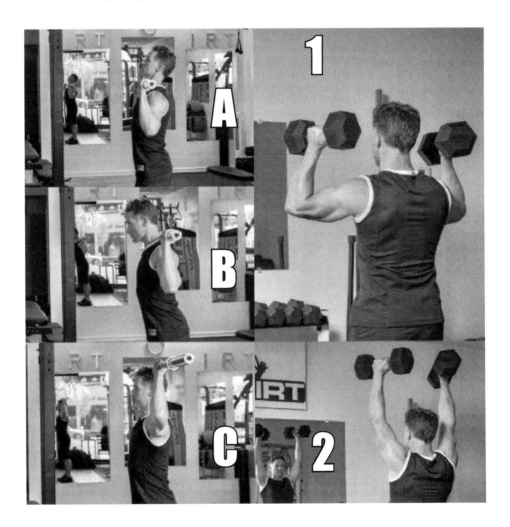

As you can see the dumbbells allow for coming down slightly lower without contacting your head or having to move out of neutral neck alignment (pictures 1 and 2).

With the single cable lat pulldown, you must either move your head backwards (photograph A) or forward (photograph B) to avoid stopping short of making contact with your head (photograph C).

**Straight Bar Lat Pulldown
Not Preferred**

**Independent Cable Pulldown
Preferred Method**

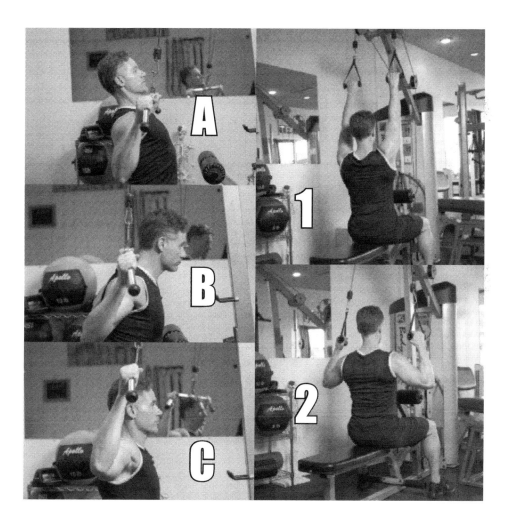

The independent cables allow for coming down lower without contacting your head (pictures 1 and 2).

When you look at the traditional barbell deadlift depicted in photographs A, B and C, the path of motion at the top (Photograph A) and bottom (Photograph C) changes slightly and the middle (Photograph B) changes greatly to avoid the bars contact with knees.

Barbell Deadlift   **Hex Bar Deadlift**
Not Preferred   **Preferred Method**

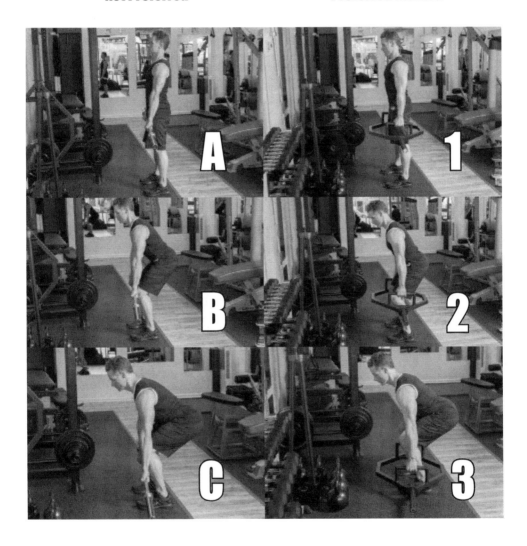

When you look at the hex bar squat pattern/deadlift, the hex is literally designed to work around the body. There is no accommodation of the body for the bar at bottom (photograph 3), top (photograph 1) or middle (photograph 2) of squat pattern.

In general, I want you to spend more time lifting weight and less time learning complex exercise maneuvers. The key is always performing the cleanest major movement pattern, whether it's with the latest exercise gadget or the most traditional exercise equipment. If the equipment hinders your exercise, use something else better suited to facilitate the movement pattern. If you are working your legs and most of the focus is on arm position, arm motion, arm speed or arm fatigue, then your exercise modality or style is taking priority over your health and fitness. If you're in a fitness competition, then this could be a necessity. However, IRT always puts your natural movement pattern first, not the modality you use. Simply perform exercises with weight that is appropriate for your body in a way that makes sense, like squatting, pulling or pushing with aligned Core Posture and listen to your body throughout the process.

IRT Principle Six:
Intrinsic Cardio and Recovery

IRT builds cardiovascular fitness in each circuit.

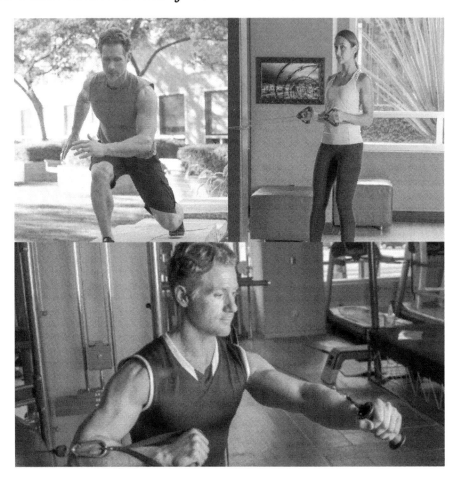

As mentioned in principle four, IRT utilizes a squatting movement, pulling movement and a pushing movement for each circuit. The beauty of performing exercises in a circuit is that you not only get active recovery (one group of muscles recovers while another group of muscles is actively working), but you increase your anaerobic and aerobic condition. Forcing blood from one major muscle group to another challenges your heart to work harder.

This means that IRT increases your cardiovascular fitness. It's important to remember that we are talking about general aerobic fitness here. If one wants to develop an optimal state of cardiovascular fitness, then see the Supplemental Cardio section and really work on whatever activity that you want to improve. Look at that as a skill set. If you want to run a marathon, practice doing that, but IRT will give you an amazing baseline to compliment any activity you love.

With IRT you will also experience similar benefits to an activity like sprinting, an example of anaerobic training. This is similar to the popular concept of HIIT training or High Intensity Interval Training.

The major difference with IRT is that the intensity is varied and channeled into very specific major movement patterns that allow you to maintain your breathing pattern, work on ideal Core Posture and target the major muscle systems of your body.

The circuit aspect of IRT is sometimes referred to as VIIT or Varied Intensity Interval Training and is what actually happens to most HIIT programs. This is because it is impossible to maintain high intensity training for long periods of time. Go sprint as fast as you can and see how long it lasts if you need proof of this.

Again, the goal should always be quality over quantity and this includes the quality of your intensity. Your focus needs to be on creating an efficient body within and also outside the workout. You are basically setting your body up to burn more calories after your workout by taking advantage of the afterburn effect. In simple terms, it means that your body will continue to burn extra calories for up to four hours after a workout.

Also, consistent exercise will increase your metabolism and, over time, make it relatively more efficient. As you gain strength by building more muscle mass and lose body fat, you'll find that the muscle is burning more calories than its counterpart in body fat. This is why IRT is about more than just burning calories in a workout. Instead it's about making your body a more productive system for all the hours of your life.

Examples of specific IRT circuits will be provided and explained in the exercise section.

Supplemental Cardio + Recovery

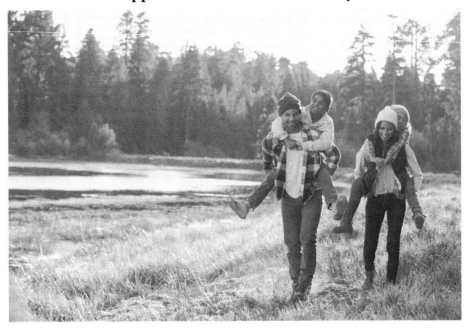

You have a great opportunity to continue your efforts on the days you don't do IRT with activities like walking, jogging, or even sprinting. The ability to walk, jog or perform appropriate sprints for your fitness level should be available to each person for as long as possible. When IRT is performed correctly it will complement and enhance all other physical activities in your life. Remember in doing your cardio that the same rules apply when it comes to breathing, posture and listening to your body.

It's a good idea to get a little something in each day, even for your rest day. Don't forget that quality trumps quantity every time. If you can only do three quality sprints, only do three. If you're not feeling up to sprinting one day, then decrease the speed and do what you can. Also, be aware that jogging and sprinting is all relative. A "jog" for one person may end up being a fast walk and their "sprint" may be walking up a hill. Do what elevates your heart rate. Your heart doesn't care what that activity is, as long as you make it a healthy option for your body.

On the seventh day of the week (when you are not doing IRT or cardio) you should recover. That doesn't mean that on that day you turn into a couch potato. It's still good to take a walk in the park, on the beach, around the block or a mall or play outside with your kids. You get the picture. Get up and move. If you live a sedentary lifestyle working at computers and sitting for long periods of time, it is even more crucial to get moving whenever you can.

Eventually as your health and fitness levels improve, you may naturally include more physical activity on your recovery day. As your level of fitness increases, increase the intensity of your walking days as well, incorporating a mixture of walking and fast-walking or hiking up a hill. It all depends on your fitness goals, how you feel and what your body is telling you. Specific options are listed below. Remember, recovery is essential to your health and wellness. Getting enough sleep will not only help you reduce stress, but it is literally when results happen. Take time to relax, keep perspective, and stay balanced when it comes to taking the appropriate time to rest.

Supplemental Cardio Practical Sidebar

Walk Days: easy comfortable pace, building towards moderate pace (pick one)

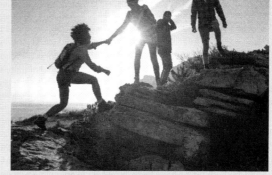

20-minute walk
30-minute walk
40-minute walk
50-minute walk
60-minute walk

Jog Days: fast walk, slow to moderate jog depending on comfort level (pick one)

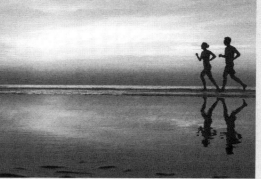

10-minute jog or fast walk
15-minute jog or fast walk
20-minute jog or fast walk
25-minute jog or fast walk
30-minute jog or fast walk

Sprint Days: fast jog to slow sprint/only hitting top speed when warmed up and confident (pick one). This could also be a hill walk or a relatively tough walk, depending on your preference and fitness level .

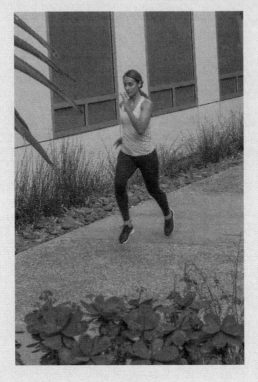

3 X 15-30 second fast jogs; 3 X 40 second rests
4 X 20-30 second fast jogs; 4 X 35 second rests
5 X 25 second runs; 5 X 30 second rests
6 X 20 second runs; 6 X 40 second rests
7 X 15 second runs; 7 X 30 second rests
8 X 10 second sprints; 8 X 30 second rests
9 X 10-15 second sprints; 9 X 30-40 second rests
10 X 10-20 second sprints; 10 X 40 second rests

Again, in all of the supplemental cardio choices as in the IRT days, it is important to listen to your body and make appropriate choices. With the high emphasis on listening to your body physically, it should be no surprise that it's just as important to listen to your body when it comes to nutrition. What follows are the nutrition guidelines for Intrinsic Nutrition that will help you know what to listen for and what questions to ask yourself.

The nutrition section has been approved by Registered Dietitian, Carrie Gabriel.

Carrie Gabriel is a food savvy dietitian who has dedicated her life to helping guide others up the stairway to overall health and wellness. She received a masters in nutritional science from California State University-Los Angeles and also has a bachelors degree in broadcast journalism and mass communication from the University of Colorado at Boulder-Colorado. She began her nutrition career working at St. Johns Hospital in Santa Monica as a nutrition aide and also worked for HealthCare Partners Medical Group as a health educator specializing in diabetes education, but later decided she wanted to gear her focus more towards preventative nutrition via private consulting, nutrition seminars, cooking demos and grocery shopping trips.

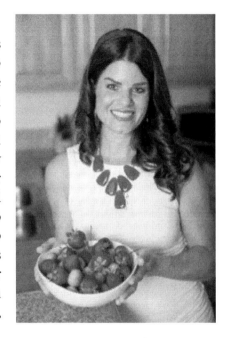

Currently, Carrie works as a freelance consulting dietitian, doing online consulting for RISE Health Coaching, conducting nutrition education seminars, cooking demonstrations and counseling for Wellness Corporate Solutions, Health Fax and Health Fitness, all companies which specialize in corporate seminars and cholesterol screenings.

Carrie's philosophy on food is the more simple and unprocessed the ingredients in a meal are the better off YOU are. She believes in the power of eating real food and enjoying what you love in moderation! She doesn't believe that weight loss can be sustained by gimmicky trends and wants to show her clients that healthy food doesn't have to be ugly, boring or taste bad. It also doesn't have to take forever to prepare! Carrie specializes in teaching her clients how to make easy, quick and healthy meals when you are pinched for time and how to understand food labels and make proper choices at the grocery store.

You can find some of Carrie's blogs and healthy, delicious recipes on Instagram, Twitter and her website, www.steps2nutrition.com.

IRT Principle Seven:

Intrinsic Nutrition Fuels Results

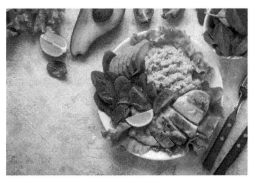

What you eat is just as important as how you work out, but much like fitness routines, nutrition has gotten convoluted to the point where most people have no idea what they should and shouldn't be eating. Intrinsic Nutrition reintroduces what should come naturally, training you to eat in a way that supports your long-term health and fitness.

Just like you may not be lifting the same amount of weight as the person next to you at the gym, you most likely will not eat the exact same diet as them. However, there are general guidelines that will benefit everyone and IN will further clarify and add specific suggestions. In getting a little more specific, IN helps you practice listening to your body and cater to your own personal nutritional needs.

Start paying attention to what you eat and how you feel before, during and after you eat. It's better to focus on what you should be eating to improve your health and wellness, and avoid focusing on what you can't eat or get hung up on fad diets that are simply unrealistic and unsustainable. If you are not sure if something is having a negative impact on your body, please see a qualified professional to help you get answers.

Intrinsic Nutrition Guidelines

I've specifically made these guidelines instead of strict principles, as this is an evolving process and there is no, one-size-fits-all approach to nutrition. What works best is consistently sticking to the guidelines that you discover are most effective for you. The six general guidelines are as follows:

1. Drink enough water.
2. Eat whole foods.
3. Cut down on (or cut out) processed foods.
4. Eat within a twelve-hour window of time.
5. Eat mindfully.
6. Make a plan and stick to it.

IN Guideline One:
Drink enough water

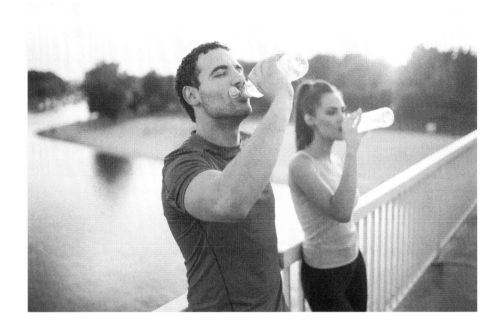

Water makes up nearly seventy percent of total body weight. It's in our bones, tissues, cells and blood. It helps to dissolve nutrients, helps metabolic reactions, lubricates joints, regulates temperature and is an important dietary source of several minerals. Hydration is vital if you want to be healthy. Water is cheap, calorie-free and supports a healthy body. Have access to water and drink it at regular intervals throughout the day.

Specifics for water

If you barely drink water, start by getting in at least thirty ounces (1L) and see how you feel. Try to work up to ninety ounces (3L) as you feel that it is needed. Always listen to your body and adjust accordingly. Also, if you eat a lot of vegetables and fruits, you may not need as much water.

Specifics for veggies, fruits and "wet" carbs

Veggies and fruit (in their raw form) have a greater percentage of water in them than other foods. They're great for hydration purposes, tend to be low in calories and high in many crucial vitamins, minerals and fiber.

Specific examples are as follows:

Percentage of water in fruits, per volume

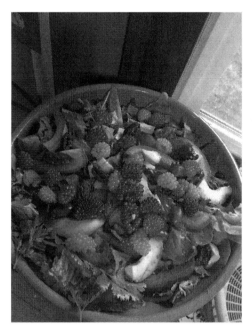

Watermelon 92
Strawberries 92
Grapefruit 91
Cantaloupe 90
Peaches   88
Pineapple   87
Cranberries 87
Oranges   87
Raspberries 87

Percentage of water in vegetables, per volume
Zucchini   95
Radish   95
Celery   95
Tomato   94
Green cabbage   93
Cauliflower   92
Eggplant   92
Red cabbage   92
Peppers   92
Spinach   92

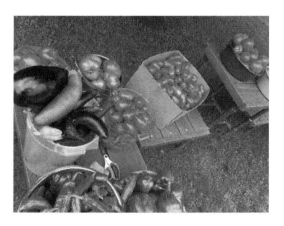

In general, "wet" carbohydrates like cooked grains and legumes have a decent amount of water in them too. Foods higher in fat on the other hand have low water content.

IN Guideline Two
Eat whole foods

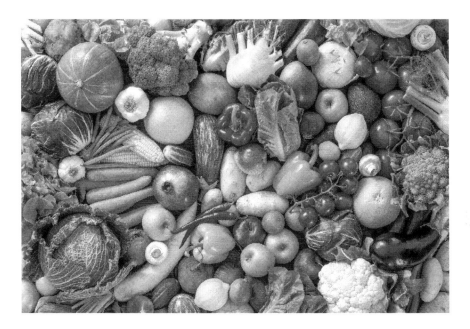

Whole foods have more nutritional value per calorie and burn more calories when you eat them than their processed counterparts. They have more fiber and are not plagued with ingredients that lead to weight gain and disease like refined sugar, refined carbohydrates, unhealthy trans-fats and artificial ingredients. Chemically processed foods can be addictive and often lead to over-consumption, resulting in weight gain and disease.

Eat foods closest to the natural state they came from--off the vine, from the ground or right from the animal. Cherries instead of cherry juice. Chicken breast instead of chicken nuggets. Potatoes instead of potato chips. Buckwheat instead of bread. Whole milk instead of skim. You get the picture.

Specific alternatives to dairy milk can include almond, coconut, hemp milk or rice milk. Be mindful of the sugars that can be added to some of these milks and look to buy them unsweetened. If you have issues with gluten, there are some excellent foods that are naturally gluten free. Quinoa and sweet potatoes are great options to use as a gluten free carbohydrate. Edamame and lentil based pasta alternatives are also excellent gluten-based pasta substitutions.

I recommend that you focus on lean proteins (grass-fed and organic if you can), vegetables, fruits and healthy fats. It is a balanced diet of these components that will best support your health and fitness.

If you're vegetarian or vegan, you can get protein from sources like chia seeds, quinoa, nuts, tempeh, etc.

Try eating a balance of proteins, fats and vegetables at every meal. Doing so will keep you satiated. Again, eat whole foods as much as possible. If you must eat packaged foods, aim for ingredient labels with five ingredients or less. If you can't pronounce it or don't know what it is, it's likely it shouldn't be going into your body.

IN Guideline Three
Cut down on or, better yet, cut out processed foods
(And this means sugar!)

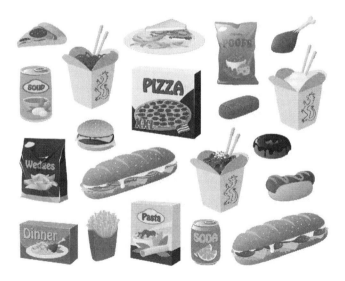

Most food is processed to some degree, but I'm talking here about chemically processed foods as opposed to mechanically processed foods. Many people don't realize how much of their diet is processed and includes preservatives, colors, textures and chemical flavors.

These additives can be addicting and have little nutritional value.

Sugar is a highly addictive substance and eating too much of it affects your teeth, liver, hormones, brain, and can lead to metabolic syndrome and even cancer. Sugar is a major cause of inflammation, which leads to diminished health in almost every capacity.

Chances are, you're eating more sugar than you realize, even if you're not gorging on candy bars or cupcakes. Sugar is added to everything from "natural" marinara sauce to "healthy" whole grain bread. Read labels and you'll be surprised how one soft drink or even a "healthy" Greek yogurt can have a full day's worth of sugar in it. Eat healthy fruits to cut that sweet tooth.

Learn what is in your food. According to the American Heart Association (AHA), the maximum amount of added sugars you should eat in a day is:

Men: 150 calories per day (37.5 grams or 9 teaspoons).
Women: 100 calories per day (25 grams or 6 teaspoons).

What is the difference between processed and natural sugar?

Processed sugar is scientifically named sucrose and found in white table sugar, cookies, candy bars, fruit drinks and even bread and chips! It is totally devoid of nutrients, has added chemicals and raises blood sugar levels faster. Yes, it can give you quick energy, but your blood sugar levels shoot up and down rapidly, leaving you hungrier than you were before you ingested it.

Even worse is high fructose corn syrup. To help you realize how bad this is for you, I'm going to get technical here. As part of the chemical process used to make high fructose corn syrup, the glucose and fructose — which are naturally bound together — become separated. This allows the fructose to mainline directly into your liver, which turns on a factory of fat production in your liver called lipogenesis, which leads to fatty liver. This, in turn, can lead to pre-diabetes and Type 2 diabetes. That's why high fructose corn syrup can be considered a real driver of the current epidemic of heart attacks, strokes, cancer, dementia and, of course, Type 2 diabetes. Simply do yourself a favor and avoid high fructose corn syrup whenever possible.

Natural sugar is something all plants produce as a byproduct of photosynthesis. Fruits and vegetables have sugar in the form of fructose, which is broken down more slowly by the body than sucrose. In addition, fruits and veggies have vitamins, minerals and fiber to slow down the digestion of their natural sugars, which leads to more stable blood sugar levels.

IN Guideline Four
Eat within a twelve-hour window.

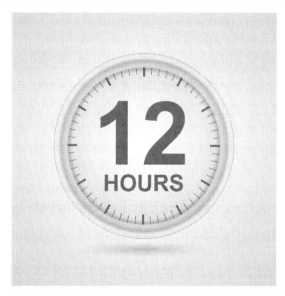

I recommend eating three to five small meals a day within a twelve-hour window of time. This is a simple way to avoid huge fluctuations in your blood sugar levels, which helps send the right signals to your brain and keep hormone levels where you want them. This is also an easier way to not only eat the right thing, but also in the appropriate portions. Portion control is also key to keeping your body working smoothly and generally is a byproduct of eating healthy at the right time.

Leave plenty of time between dinner at night and breakfast the next morning. Doing so gives your body time to recover. Your quality of sleep will also most likely improve. Much research suggests twelve hours; though some research suggests that a gap of up to fourteen hours for women and sixteen for men can be beneficial. Remember it's only helpful if you can sustain the behavior. I recommend that you start with twelve hours and see how it works for you. Small, sustainable changes over the long term make huge differences.

IN Guideline Five
Eat mindfully

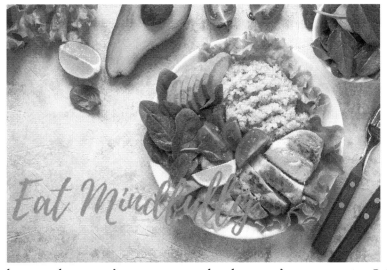

Think about what you're eating and why you're eating it. I hear so many stories of people making one poor meal choice and then feeling "damned if they do and damned if they don't." They proceed to go off the rails and eat anything and everything in sight because they feel they've already sabotaged their progress. This kind of outlook perpetuates a vicious cycle. It's okay to have a day where you know you ate too much or you're on vacation kicking back and eating whatever comes your way. To make this sustainable for the rest of your life, you will have moments like this.

The people who succeed don't let things like this propel them back into their old habits. They get right back on track, without feeling guilty or frustrated. Life happens. Enjoy the food, don't feel guilty and then get back to eating healthy foods. Usually my clients don't crave unhealthy food once they start making better decisions, and when they do go back to their old eating habits, they feel noticeably worse. That sickening feeling used to be their norm and noticing the difference is further motivation to keep eating in a healthy manner.

Sometimes the reason people eat too much or crave unhealthy foods is because their current view of "eating perfectly for their body" is skewed. In many cases, they are eating too little food for their bodies to work efficiently. This is a big one. When people end up under eating for too many days in a row, they usually get hungry and eventually overeat or binge. Instead of feeling defeated, reassess if you need to add a few more calories in at breakfast and lunch, in order not to be hungry and ready to eat anything in the late afternoon and early evening.

IN Guideline Six
Make a plan and stick to it

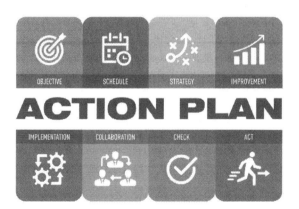

You will need to experiment to understand what works for you, but once you figure that out, stick to it. Consistently following the guidelines is key to success.

Keep the following questions in mind as you get started. Do you have more energy when you eat plant-based foods? Do you lack energy when you don't eat meat? How does sugar make you feel? Heartburn after spicy foods? How do you tolerate gluten? How does dairy make you feel? Listen to what your body is telling you.

Sample Grocery List/Cleanse

PROTEINS
3 oz. tuna, canned in water
3 oz. ahi tuna, broiled
3 oz. lean ground turkey
3 oz. boneless, skinless chicken (preferably organic), broiled
4 egg whites, scrambled
2 egg whites and 1 whole egg, scrambled
3 oz. salmon, tilapia or mahi-mahi, broiled

CARBOHYDRATES
½ cup brown rice, quinoa and/or quinoa pasta cooked in water
½ cup oatmeal or steel cut oats, cooked in water
½ sweet potato, baked
1 slice Ezekiel bread or 1 medium Ezekiel tortilla
½ cup kidney beans, black beans, garbanzo beans, etc.
drained or cooked in water if they are not the canned ones
½ cup strawberries, blueberries, raspberries or blackberries
1 apple or banana, small
Spinach, kale, arugula, ANY VEGGIE as much as you would like!
Preferably green and raw, but can be sautéed lightly in olive oil.

FATS
2 tbsp. natural peanut or almond butter
2 tbsp. extra virgin olive oil
¼ cup raw almonds or walnuts
¼ cup hempseeds or flaxseeds
¼ avocado
¼ cup sunflower or pumpkin seed

ENJOY THESE CONDIMENTS AND SPICES AT YOUR LEISURE
(Let your condiments compliment your food, not overpower it.)

Organic Mustard and Ketchup, Braggs Liquid Amino Acids, Balsamic Vinegar, Salsa, Mrs. Dash, Vanilla and/or Almond extracts, Cinnamon, Ginger, Garlic, Lemon Pepper, Cayenne, Cilantro, Parsley, Mint, Basil, Stevia, Low Sodium Chicken or Vegetable Broth, Plain/Reduced Sodium Tomato Sauce/Paste, Flavor God seasonings

IRT & IN
It's always a good idea to check with a doctor before you make any major changes to your diet and exercise.

For sustainable health and fitness results it is always advisable to combine healthy eating and appropriate exercise, since diet and exercise complement one another.

Take Intrinsic Resistance Training and Intrinsic Nutrition, apply them and learn more about how you respond to each exercise and enjoy the food you eat. IRT is about balance and it sets you up for long term success. If you've read this far, I know you have the perseverance, knowledge and personal accountability it will take to succeed. Enjoy your journey and make sure your health and fitness always supports you getting out and doing everything you want to in life.

FINAL THOUGHTS
Having spent so much time in the fitness industry, I have had to constantly remind myself and explain to my clients why to stick to a refined version of the basics that work and not embrace every latest fitness fad. Believe me, it would have been easier in the short term to succumb to the pressure, though senseless in the long term. I returned to the industry at an exciting time in the early 2000's. As sound science and technique helped me recover from self-inflicted injuries, mainstream fitness was headed in a different direction. In the Twenty-First-Century, the fitness industry has experienced greater freedom infused with endless

intensity. This combination misses the mark for purposes of general health and wellness. However, if you harness and direct this new potential with the general IRT principles outlined, you will benefit from the updated science in its appropriate context. I hope this provides you the specific resources to judge for yourself what is effective practice. The goal is to get out and enjoy life, not turn your life into a workout. Intrinsic Resistance Training is a means to that end.

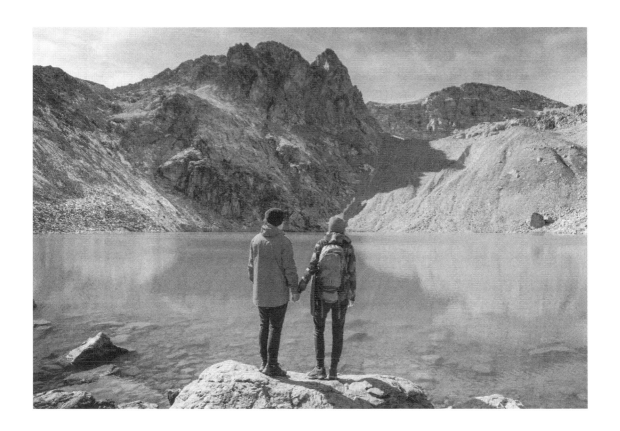

IRT Practical Application

Before we look at the specific individual exercise options and sample workouts, please remember the bigger picture of squat, pull and push patterns when deciding to include or exclude exercises from your workout. The samples below are only that. Don't let them or the sample workouts limit your options in any way. Instead let them help inform what other similar options you want to add in the future.

Squat Pattern:

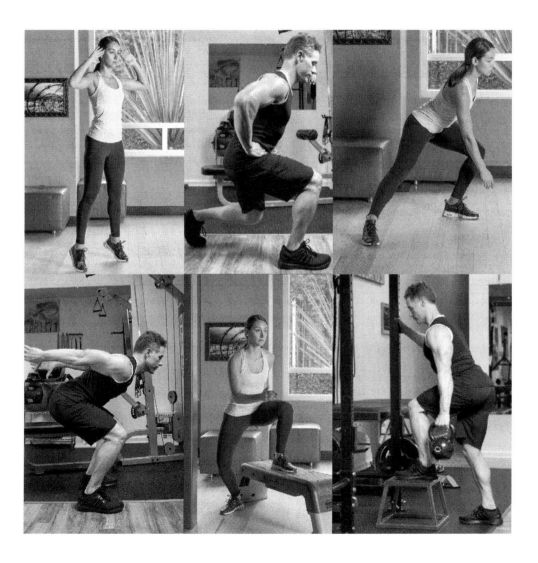

Pull Pattern:

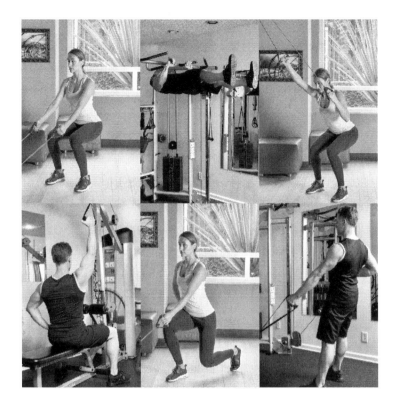

Push Pattern:

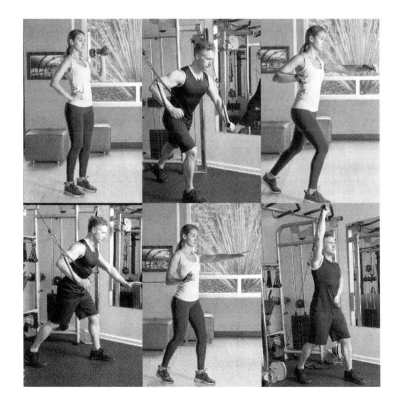

With these options in mind, we'll get even more specific. If your own primary workout will be at home, please proceed to the home workout section after your warm up. If your primary workout will be in the gym, please proceed to the gym workout after your warm up. Remember that each of these sections should complement the other. If you are a gym goer and find yourself on vacation with no gym, the home workout will be a great supplement while on vacation. Also, if you work out at home primarily and you find yourself at a gym on a guest pass or even decide to join up, you'll be no stranger to the major movement patterns.

THE IRT WARM UP FOR GYM & HOME WORKOUTS

In this section, I'm going to show you specific warm up exercises for both the gym and home setting.

Sample Warm Up

Step 1: The Warm Up/ Body Check

Every workout should start with specific exercises that allow you to assess your baseline Core Posture and give you an opportunity to reinforce stability and mobility in the appropriate areas. If you're like most people, you have muscle imbalances. You've also probably spent a good portion of the day sitting or driving with less than ideal posture. Getting on a treadmill and walking for five minutes will probably reinforce that posture and those imbalances and it's not recommended here. Instead, follow this general plan to combat the basic postural issues brought about by a sedentary lifestyle through reinforcing and activating long spine Core Posture.

One more thing I want to mention here that pertains to all the exercises in the book. Pay particular attention to your form. Compare how you look to the photos here to check your body alignment. I would rather have you do one rep using correct posture than five reps with your body twisted in the wrong direction. Appropriate form provides the best chance of attaining the full benefit of the exercise.

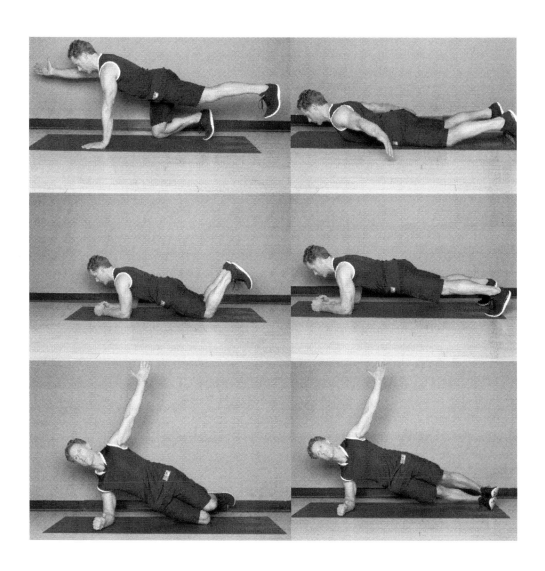

1. "Quadriplex"

Position 1: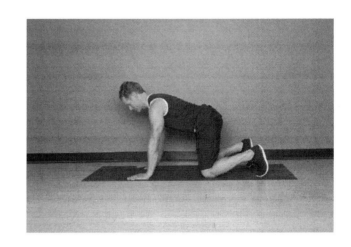

Position 2: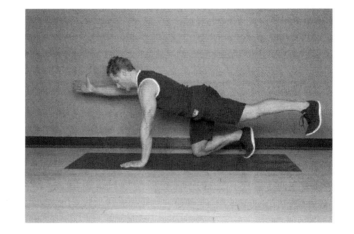

Position 3: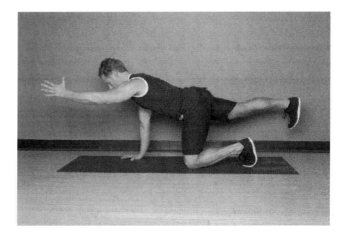

84

What it works: The Quadriplex is meant to check/activate your Core Posture anti-rotation by mobilizing your hips and shoulders. The idea is not to twist your body. Again, any extra movement is counterproductive to the goal of the exercise.

How to do it: Kneel on all fours in a table-top position and breathe in to stabilize your Core Posture. Slowly lift one arm at a time off the ground and extend it in front of you with your thumb up until your arm is parallel with the ground. If this feels stable, alternate your arms. Once that feels stable, try your legs. Extend your leg back behind you, foot flexed, as if you were going to kick something with your heel until your whole leg is parallel to the ground and your torso. The goal is to move the hip/leg without changing or compromising the position of your spine/torso. Do this on both legs and then do the opposing arm and leg together at the same time.

Perform: 1-2 sets of 10 repetitions (5 on each side).

2. "Prone Cobra"

Position 1:

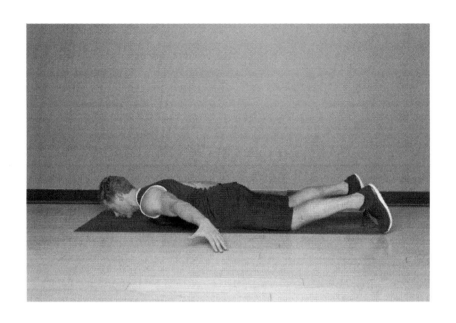

Position 2:

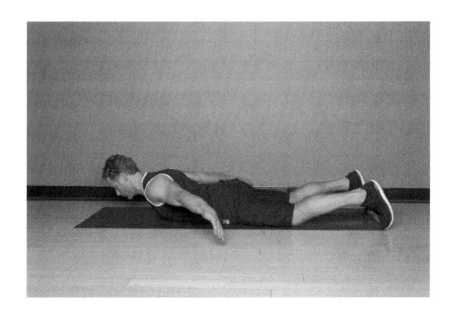

What it works: The Prone Cobra mobilizes the upper back and external rotators of the shoulders and stabilizes the neck in a neutral position.

How to do it: Lie face down on the floor, tuck your chin in as if you could hold a grapefruit or softball between your chin and collarbones. Remember to continue thinking long spine. As you raise your upper chest off the ground, pull the shoulder blades down and back and around the ribs and rotate your thumbs away from your body towards the ceiling. Hold for a second, return to the start position with your hands palm down slightly away from your body and repeat exercise. Remember that you shouldn't feel too much work in your neck or lower back. If you do, reassess your form and start over or rest.

Perform: 1-2 sets of 10 reps.

3. A. "Plank"

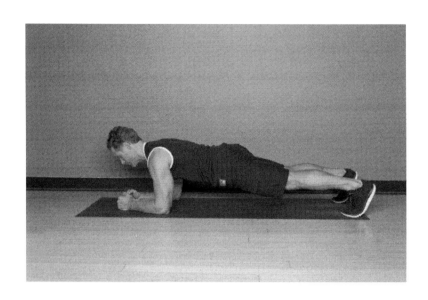

3. B. "Modified Plank"

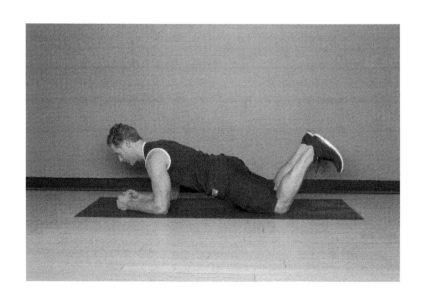

What it works (3A): The "Plank" is meant to stabilize your Core Posture by checking/ activating your anti-extension (don't arch).

How to do it: Lie down facing the floor with your forearms on the mat and your feet up on the balls of your toes. Keep your spine long and neutral. Do not over-arch your back. Hold your body steady for ten seconds, then release.

For beginners (3B), this exercise can be done on your knees.

Perform 1-2 sets of 10 second holds focusing on form more than holding it too long with compromised posture.

4. A. "Side Plank"

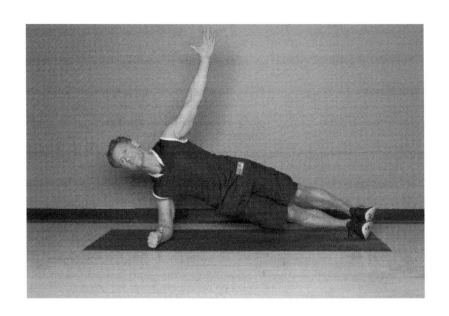

4. B. "Modified Side Plank"

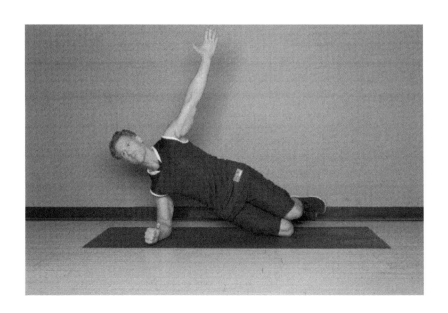

What it does (4A): The "Side Plank" is meant to stabilize your Core Posture by checking/ activating your anti-lateral flexion.

How to do it: Lie on your side with your weight resting against your forearm and the side of your foot. Place the opposite foot on top of it and raise the opposite arm in the air for balance. Again, the spine is held straight with no sideways bend.
Perform: Hold position for ten seconds, then release. Then switch sides and repeat.

For beginners (4B), this exercise can be done on the side of the knees.

5. "Kneeling Hip Flexor Stretch"

Position 1

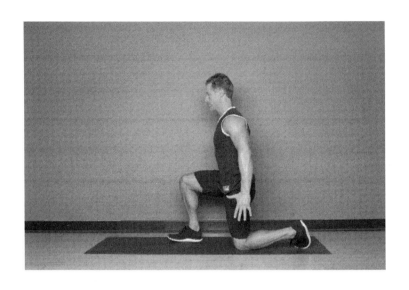

Position 2

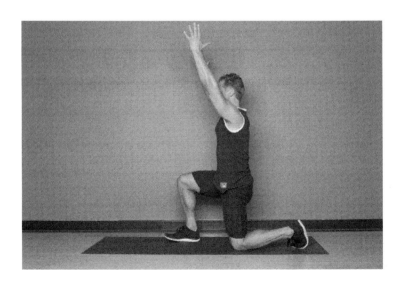

What it does: The "Kneeling Hip Flexor stretch" is meant to reinforce your Core Posture by testing your ability to maintain your neutral long spine position and mobilize each hip and both shoulders.

How to do it: Start by placing one leg in front of you, with your foot on the ground. The opposite leg is bent at the knee and the toes are flexed. Then raise both arms over your head, keeping your torso straight. Hold position then switch legs and repeat.

Perform: 1 set of 5-8 reps on each side.

Sample Gym workout:

In this section, I'm going to show you specific exercises you can do in a gym setting. At this point, you should have completed the warm up exercises. These are potential options, but you can visit the website for other options that you can substitute into the workout. The idea is to get you judging for yourself what the appropriate exercises are for you, based off of the IRT Principles and how you feel each workout.

Remember the Principles for all Exercises:

1) Listen to your body and work out mindfully. Always go for quality over quantity and know which muscle groups you're working with clean movement patterns. Never ignore or work through pain.

2) Breathing acts as your inner support for every exercise. Breathe in through the nose as the targeted major muscle group elongates and breathe out through the mouth as they shorten.

3) Posture is fundamental to every exercise and maintaining that long spine neutral posture constitutes true core work or what IRT refers to as Core Posture. Resist being pulled forward into a hunched over position, backward into an overly arched position, collapsing sideways or over rotating in either direction to ensure you maintain your optimal long spine Core Posture.

4) Foot position is the foundation to every exercise, whether you are laying, sitting or especially when standing. Maintain stable foot position. This means stand on the three main points of contact of your feet: your heel, ball of big toe, and ball of little toe. Make sure that your foot remains connected to the ground and doesn't roll or collapse in any direction.

5) Perform major movement patterns. Each main circuit should consist of a squatting, pulling and pushing movement. You will start to see similarities in exercises that at first glance seem totally different.

6) Keep it moving with cardio and take time to recover. Work out in circuits to give one muscle group time to recover as you use a fresh movement pattern to keep your heart rate at a challenging but doable pace where form doesn't suffer.

7)Proper nutrition fuels results. Look to the nutritional guidelines to support your health and fitness. You deserve the right foods at the appropriate times.

The rest of this section contains specific exercises to be performed in a typical exercise session. If you're just starting out, you'll be working on a learning phase. The guidelines for this are three sets of six repetitions.

As you become more comfortable with your sets you can add more weight and follow the general guidelines for periodization below. This will help you build up your endurance and add more tone to your muscles. When that becomes easy to do, then increase the weight for each exercise. This will build up your strength. But always, always, always pay attention to your body. It will give you clear signals for when enough is enough!

Remember the general rep schemes for learning a new exercise:

3X6 for Learning phase with light or manageable weight
3x15 for Endurance
4x10 for Hypertrophy
5x5 for Strength

Circuit Number One

1A. "Body Weight Squat"

Position 1

Position 2

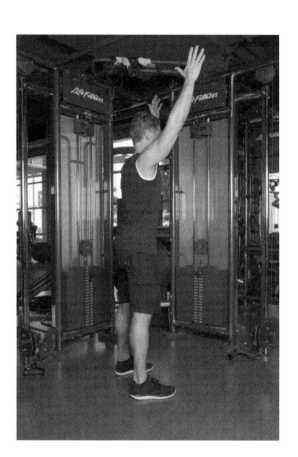

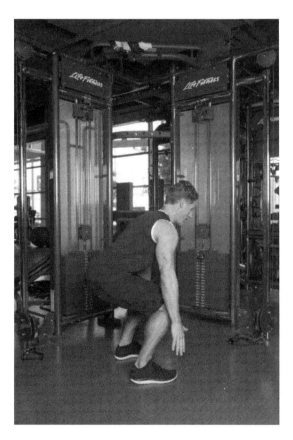

What it works: This squatting exercise works the glutes, your entire leg along with Core Posture anti-flexion (don't hunch). Make sure you stop yourself from collapsing or hunching.

How to do it: Stand with feet hip-width apart in a tripod foot position with neutral Core Posture. Breathe in as you sit back into your hips, lengthening the glute muscles. Make sure you're hinging at your hips, knees and ankles, and at the bottom of the movement take a pause. Then stand up tall, driving the hips up over your legs. Remember there is no absolute rule as to how low you should go, because everyone's body is different. Unless you're in a squatting competition, you should go down only as far as you can, performing the exercise properly.

2A. "Standing Lat Row"

Position 1

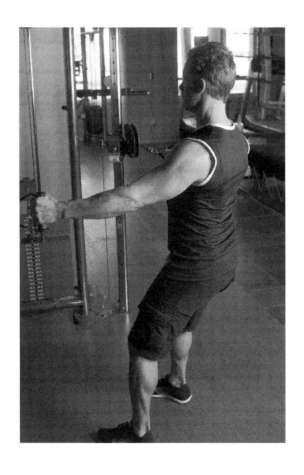

Position 2

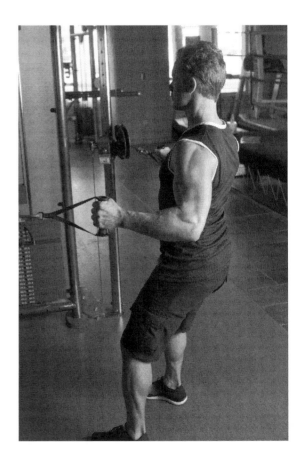

What it works: This pulling movement exercise works the lats, shoulder stability, the back part of the shoulders and the front part of the arms or biceps, along with Core posure anti-flexion (don't hunch).

How to do it: Stand facing the weight stack that you are going to pull and hunker down to counter-balance the weight. Grip the handles and initiate the exercise by stabilizing or connecting to your shoulder blades by pulling them down, back and around. Draw the elbows back to your sides maintaining long spine Core Posture. The hinge happens from the shoulder complex and the elbow while maintaining neutral wrist position.

3A. "Standing Chest Press"

Position 1

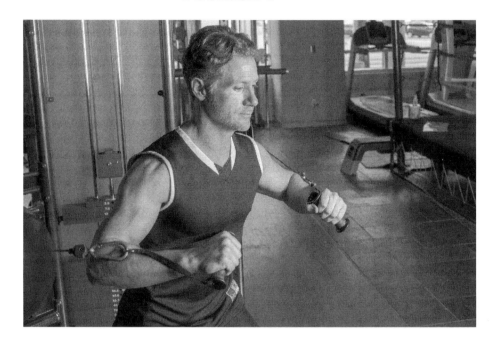

Position 2

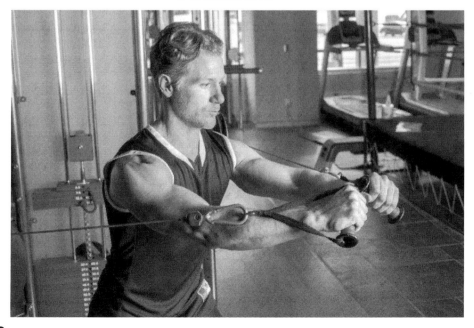

What it works: This pushing movement works the chest, front part of the shoulders and back part of the arms or triceps, along with Core posture anti-extention (don't over-arch).

How to do it: Stand facing away from the weight stack that you are going to press with a long spine posture and your whole body from trail leg to head as if you're in a plank position at about a 45-degree angle to the floor. Start the movement stabilizing and driving through the ball of the back foot by reaching with your arms out in front of you. Breathe in as you stretch your chest muscles by bending at the elbows and shoulder complex and let the elbows drop slightly down to your sides. When you get to about 90 degrees, hold and then exhale, driving the movement from your chest by bringing your inner elbows together.

Circuit Number Two

1B. "Step Up"

Position 1

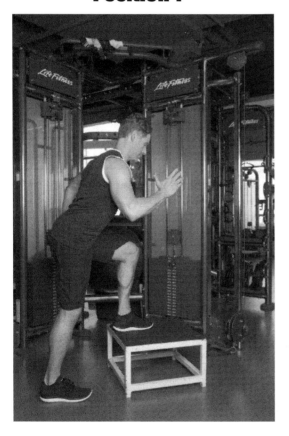

Position 2

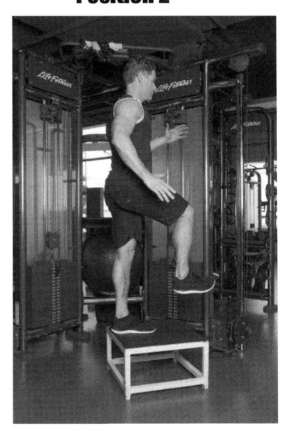

What it works: This exercise works the glutes, your entire leg along with Core Posture anti-lateral flexion (don't sway sideways). The goal is to keep your body straight without hunching or bending sideways.

How to do it: Stand facing a step or secure elevated surface. Start at a height low enough to maintain your Core Posture and hinge at the hip knee and ankle. Begin by putting one foot up on the step-in tripod foot position, while the other foot is on the ground. The foot on the step is the working leg and you will start your first repetition by breathing in and holding for a second. Next exhale as you drive the hip up over the leg. You will be standing tall and your glute muscles will shorten. Then sit back into that same hip as you breathe in and the glutes elongate. Repeat and remember to keep most of your weight on the step at all times.

2B. "One Arm Lat Row"

Position 1

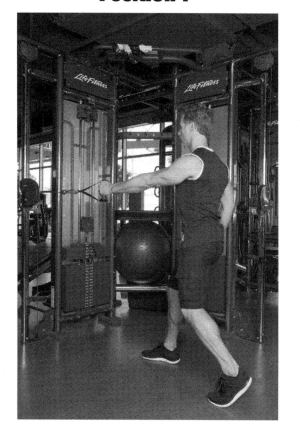

Position 2

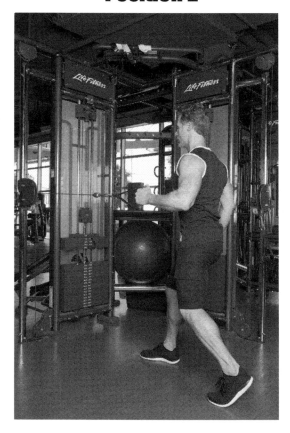

What it works: This pulling movement works the lats and corresponding arm along with Core Posture anti-rotation (don't twist). Again, maintain straight body posture without giving in to the tendency to twist.

How to do it: Stand facing the weight stack you are going to pull in a split stance, which means opposite leg forward to the arm that you're pulling with. Grab the handle. When you feel comfortable, place most of the weight on the front leg and breathe in and activate your Core Posture anti-rotation. Initiate the movement by stabilizing your shoulder blades by pulling them down, back and around, and then breathe out as you draw your arm back by your side. Hold for a second and then breathe in as you release the cable back to the starting position and repeat.

3B. "Modified Push Up"

Position 1

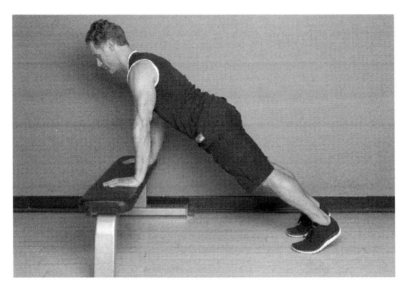

Position 2

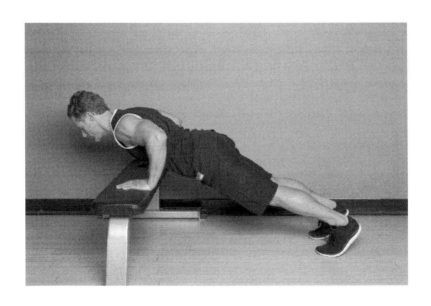

What it works: This pushing movement targets the chest, front part of the shoulders and back part of the arms along with Core Posture anti-extension (don't over-arch).

How to do it: Use any surface elevated up off the ground, be it bar, bench, platform or even a wall. Place your hands shoulder width apart and extend your arms out perpendicular to your body and activate your Core Posture anti-extension. Arms should be extended, but not locked. Slowly lower yourself, bending at the elbows and shoulders, keeping your wrists neutral until your elbows and shoulders are at about 90 degrees as you breathe in and stretch your chest muscles. Hold for a second at the bottom, and then breathe out as your chest muscles shorten and drive you back up.

Circuit Number Three

1C. "Hip Hinge"

Position 1   Position 2

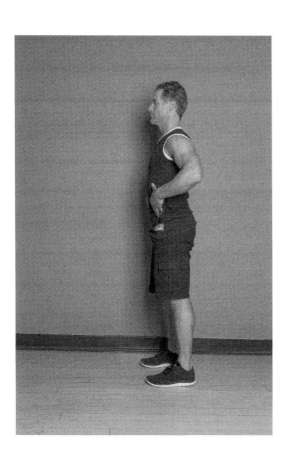 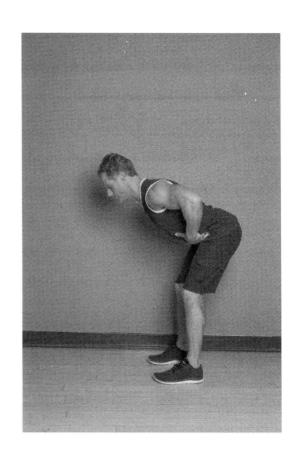

*Although "Hip Hinge" is not a Squat Pattern, the ability to mobilize your hips while maintaining neutral long spine Core Posture is essential to loaded movement. I therefore include it here as a part of this major circuit.

What it works: The hip hinge is meant to target the hip complex, which stretches your glutes and hamstrings and also challenges your Core Posture anti-flexion (don't hunch).

How to do it: Stand with hands on your ribs and top of pelvis to ensure that your torso doesn't move or flex or extend. Your hand position should not change. Hinging only at your hips, stick the butt out and let the hips travel backwards. Do not hunch your back. The knees should be straight, but not locked. Avoid changing the knee position during each repetition.

Like with any of these exercises as you progress and feel comfortable, you can add weight to the movement patterns. Please remember to add weight in small increments and listen to your body.

3C. "Standing high alternating arms Lat Row"

Position 1 and 3

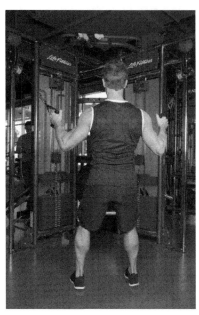

Position 2

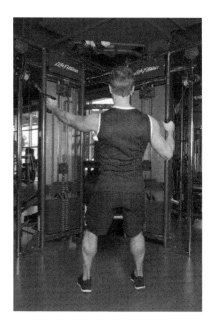

Position 4

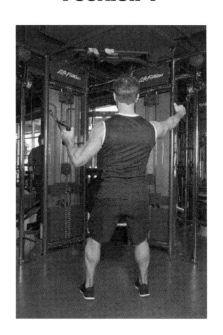

What it works: This pulling movement works the lats, middle and lower traps, rhomboids, rear delts and biceps. Alternating the arms gives you an anti-rotation (don't twist) Core Posture demand.

How to do it: Stand hunkered down facing the weight you are going to pull. With a firm grip on the handles stand straight with the spine neutral. Initiate the movement by pulling the shoulder blades down, back and around to engage the lats. Move the elbows back next, keeping the forearms parallel to the cables. Once you're holding in position 2, you can start extending one arm out and then return that arm fully to the second position and then switch to the other arm. Resist the tendency to twist your body.

3C. "One Arm Decline Press"

Position 1

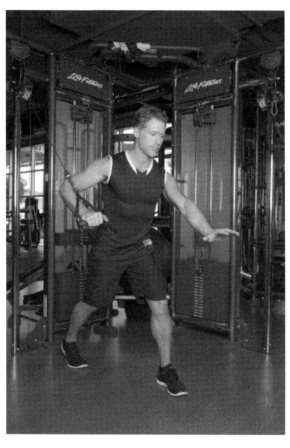

Position 2

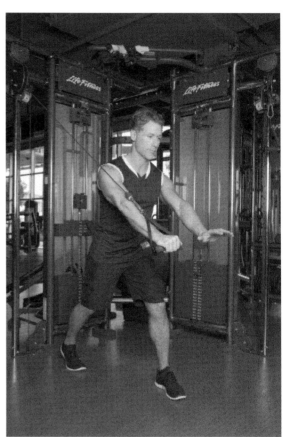

What it works: This pushing movement is designed to emphasize the chest, front delts and triceps along with Core Posture anti-rotation (don't twist).

How to do it: Facing away from the resistance, place yourself in a stable split stance. The opposite foot to the arm that you're pushing with is forward. Think about the dynamics of a two-arm regular chest press to guide you to the right position. Keep your body square and weight driven off of the back leg from the ball of the foot. Start with both arms extended in front of you. Pretend your empty hand is pushing something to help stabilize that side and as you bring the loaded arm back, stretching your chest muscles, breathe in. Hold for a second and then breathe out as you drive the hand back to center line returning the chest muscles to a shortened position.

Sample Home Workout:

In this section, I'm going to show you specific exercises you can do at home or in almost any other location, for that matter. At this point, you should have completed the warm up exercises.

With these exercises, you're replicating the same movements as you do in the gym workout by using resistance bands and dumbbells instead of machines. I have seen many clients get amazing results doing this at home. These are potential options, but you can visit the website for other options that you can substitute into the workout. The idea is to get you judging for yourself what the appropriate exercises are for you, based off of the IRT Principles and how you feel each workout.

What You Need:
-Resistance bands
-Dumbbells
-Step

Optional:
-Door mounted band unit

Remember the Principles for all Exercises:

1) Listen to your body and work out mindfully. Always go for quality over quantity and know which muscle groups you're working with clean movement patterns. Never ignore or work through pain.

2) Breathing acts as your inner support for every exercise. Breathe in through the nose as the targeted major muscle group elongates and breathe out through the mouth as they shorten.

3) Posture is fundamental to every exercise and maintaining that long spine neutral posture constitutes true core work or what IRT refers to as Core Posture. Stabilize your torso and resist being pulled forward into a hunched over position, backward into an overly arched position, collapsing sideways or over rotating in either direction to ensure you maintain your optimal long spine Core Posture.

4) Foot position is the foundation to every exercise, whether you are laying, sitting or especially when standing. Maintain a stable foot position. This means stand on the three main points of contact of your feet, your heel, (ball of) big toe, and (ball of) little toe. Make sure that your foot remains connected to the ground connection and doesn't roll or collapse in any direction.

5) Perform major movement patterns. Each main circuit should consist of a squatting, pulling and pushing movement. You will start to see similarities in exercises that at first glance seem totally different.

6) Keep it moving with cardio and take time to recover. Work out in circuits to give one muscle group time to recover as you use a fresh movement pattern to keep your heart rate at a challenging, but doable pace where form doesn't suffer.

7) Proper nutrition fuels results. Look to the nutritional guidelines to support your health and fitness. You deserve the right foods at the appropriate times.

The rest of this section contains specific exercises to be performed in a typical exercise session. If you're just starting out, you'll be working on a learning phase. The guidelines for this are three sets of six repetitions.

As you become more comfortable with your sets you can add more weight and follow the general guidelines for periodization below. This will help you build up your endurance and add more tone to your muscles. When that becomes easy to do, then increase the weight for each exercise. This will build up your strength. But always, always, always pay attention to your body. It will give you clear signals for when enough is enough!

Remember the general rep schemes for learning a new exercise:

3X6 for Learning phase with light or manageable weight
3x15 for Endurance
4x10 for Hypertrophy
5x5 for Strength

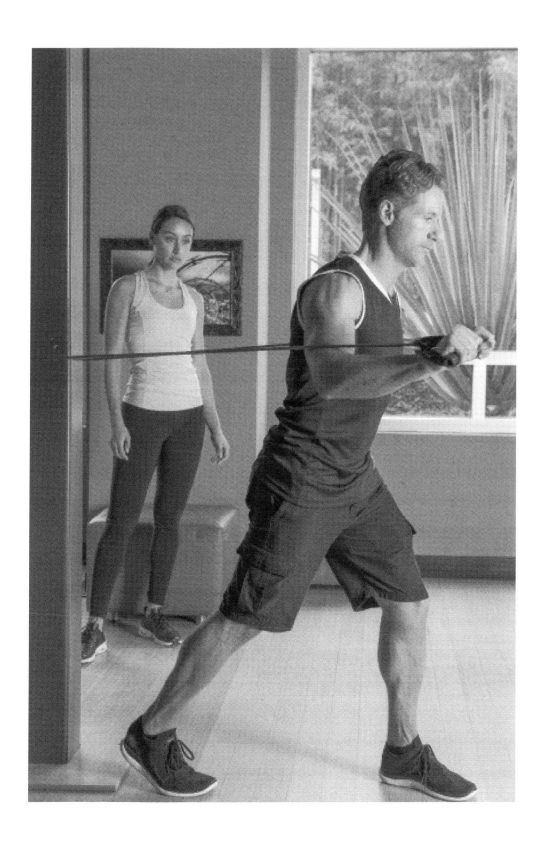

Circuit Number One

1A. "Body Weight Squat"

Position 1   **Position 2**

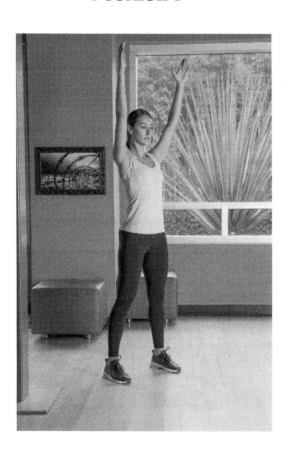
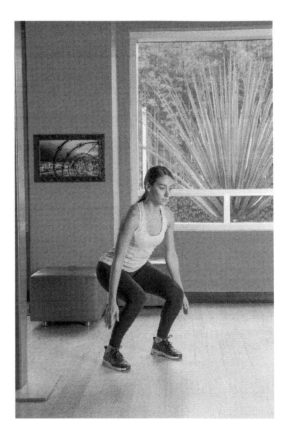

What it works: This squatting exercise works the glutes, your entire leg along with Core Posture anti-flexion (don't hunch).

How to do it: Stand with feet hip width apart in tripod foot position with neutral Core Posture. Breathe in as you sit back into your hips, lengthening the glute muscles. Make sure you're hinging at your hips, knees and ankles, and at the bottom of movement take a pause. Then stand up tall, driving the hips up over your legs. Remember there is no absolute rule as to how low you should go, because everyone's body is different. Unless you're in a squatting competition, you should go down only as far as you can, performing the exercise properly.

2A. Band Standing Lat Row

Position 1

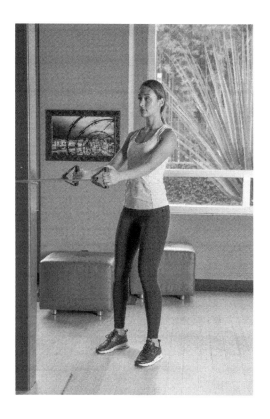

Position 2

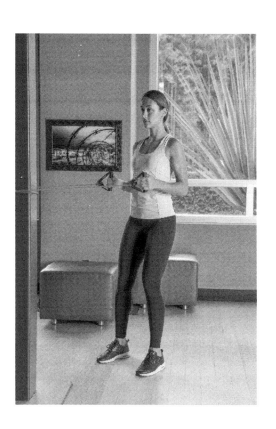

*Although "Hip Hinge" is not a Squat Pattern, the ability to mobilize your hips while maintaining neutral long spine Core Posture is essential to loaded movement. I therefore include it here as a part of this major circuit.

What it works: This pulling movement exercise works the lats, shoulder stability, the back part of the shoulders, and the front part of the arms or biceps along with Core posture anti-flexion (don't hunch).

How to do it: Secure the resistance band on the door. Stand facing the resistance that you are going to pull and hunker down to counter-balance the weight. Grip the handles and initiate the exercise by stabilizing or connecting to your shoulder blades by pulling them down, back and around. Then draw the elbows back to your sides maintaining long spine Core Posture. The hinge happens from the shoulder complex and the elbow, while maintaining neutral wrist position.

3A. Band Split-Stance Chest Press

Position 1

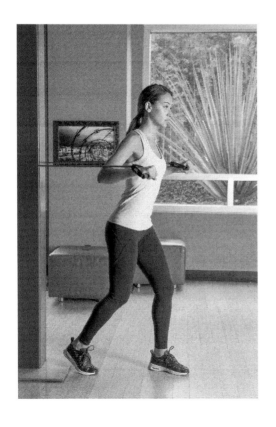

Position 2

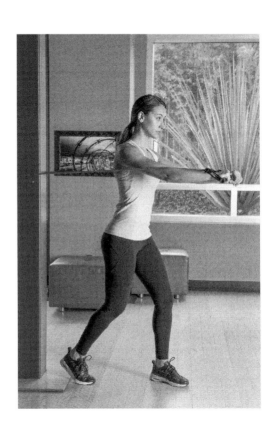

What it works: This pushing movement works the chest, front part of the shoulders, and back part of the arms or triceps, along with Core posture anti-extention (don't over-arch).

How to do it: Secure the resistance band on the door. Stand facing away from the resistance that you are going to press with a long spine posture and your whole body from trail leg to head as if you're in a plank position at about a 45-degree angle to the floor. Start the movement stabilizing and driving through the ball of the back foot by reaching with your arms out in front of you. Breathe in as you stretch your chest muscles by bending at the elbows and shoulder complex and let the elbows drop slightly down to your sides. When you get to about 90 degrees, hold and then exhale driving the movement from your chest by bringing your inner elbows together.

Circuit Number Two

1B. "Step Up"

Position 1   **Position 2**

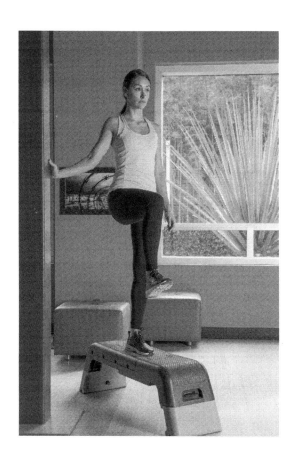 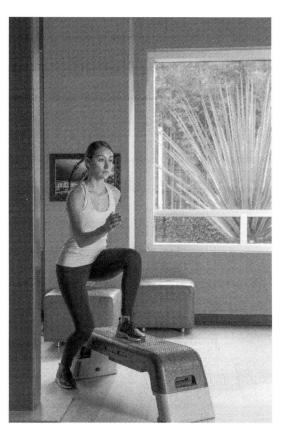

What it works: This exercise works the glutes, your entire leg along with Core Posture anti-lateral flexion (don't bend sideways).

How to do it: Stand facing a step or secure elevated surface. Start at low height where you can maintain your Core Posture and hinge at the hip knee and ankle. Begin by putting one foot up on the step-in tripod foot position, while the other foot is on the ground. The foot on the step is the working leg and you will start your first repetition by breathing in and holding for a second. Next exhale as you drive the hip up over the leg so you're standing tall and your glute muscles shorten. Then sit back into that same hip as you breathe in and the glutes elongate. Repeat and remember to keep most of your weight on the step at all times.

2B. One Arm Lat Row with Band

Position 1

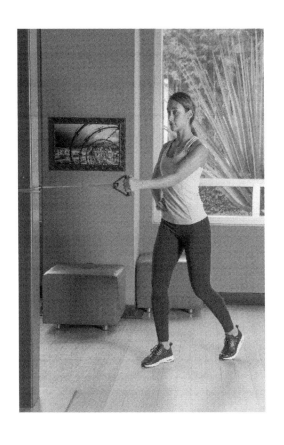

Position 2

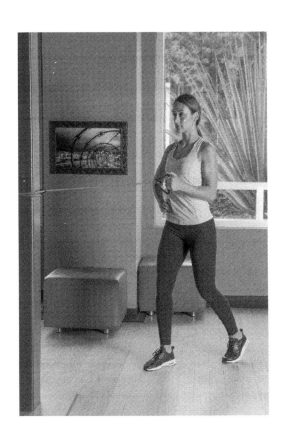

What it works: This pulling movement works the lats and corresponding arm along with Core Posture anti-rotation (don't twist).

How to do it: Secure the resistance band about waist height. Stand facing the resistance you are going to pull in a split stance (opposite leg forward to arm that you're pulling with) and grab the handle. When you feel comfortable place most of the weight on the front leg and breathe in and activate your Core Posture anti-rotation (don't twist). Initiate the movement by stabilizing your shoulder blades (pulling them down, back and around) and then breathe out as you draw your arm back by your side. Hold for a second and then breathe in as you release back to the starting position and repeat.

3B. Modified Push-Up

Position 1

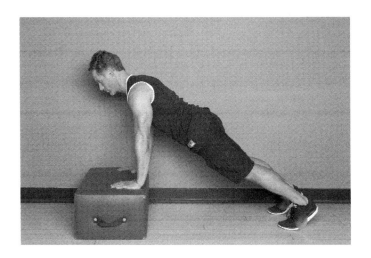

Position 2

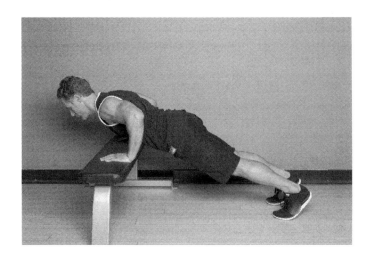

What it works: This pushing movement targets both the chest, front part of the shoulders and back part of the arms along with Core Posture anti-extension (don't over-arch).

How to do it: Use any surface elevated up off the ground, be it bar, bench, platform or even a wall. Place your hands shoulder width apart and extend your arms out perpendicular to your body and activate your Core Posture anti-extension (don't arch). Arms should be extended, but not locked. Slowly lower yourself bending at the elbows and shoulders, keeping your wrists neutral until your elbows and shoulders are at about 90 degrees as you breathe in and stretch your chest muscles. Hold for a second at the bottom and then breathe out as your chest muscles shorten and drive you back up.

Circuit Number Three

1C. Hip Hinge

Position 1

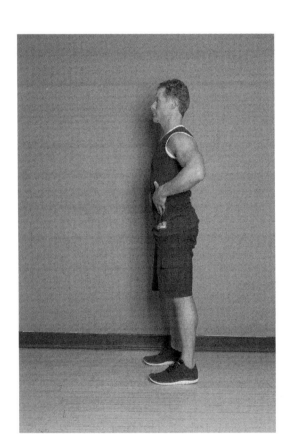

Position 2

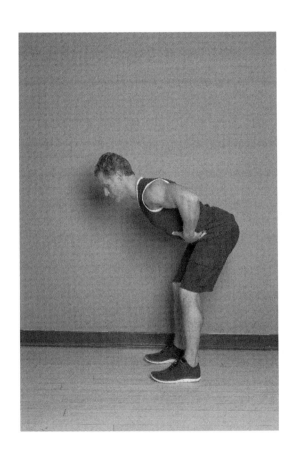

*Although "Hip Hinge" is not a Squat Pattern, the ability to mobilize your hips while maintaining neutral long spine Core Posture is essential to loaded movement. I therefore include it here as a part of this major circuit.

What it works: Your glutes and hamstrings along with Core Posture anti-flexion (don't hunch).

Stand with hands on your ribs and top of pelvis to ensure that your torso doesn't move/flex or extend (your hand position should not change) and hinging only at your hips, stick the butt out and let the hips travel backwards. The knees should be straight, but not locked. Avoid changing the knee position during each repetition.

Like with any of these exercises, as you progress and feel comfortable, you can add weight to the movement patterns. Please remember to add weight in small increments and listen to your body.

2C. Standing Lat Row with alternating arms

Positions 1 and 3

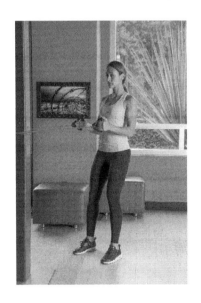

Position 2

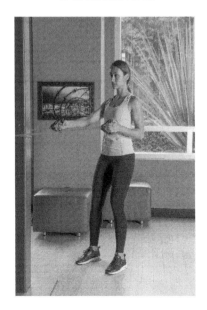

Position 4

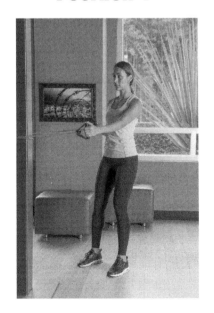

What it works: This pulling movement works the lats, middle and lower traps, rhomboids, rear delts, and biceps. Alternating the arms gives you an anti-rotation (don't twist) Core Posture demand.

How to do it: Secure the resistance band about waist height. Stand hunkered down facing the resistance you are going to pull. With a firm grip on the handles stand straight with the spine neutral. Initiate the movement by pulling the shoulder blades down and back and around to engage the lats. Move the elbows back next and keep the forearms parallel to the cables. Once you're holding in position 2, you can start by extending one arm out and returning that arm fully to the second position and then switching to the other arm.

3C. One Arm Chest Press

Position 1

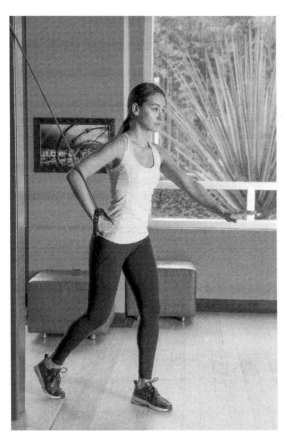

Position 2

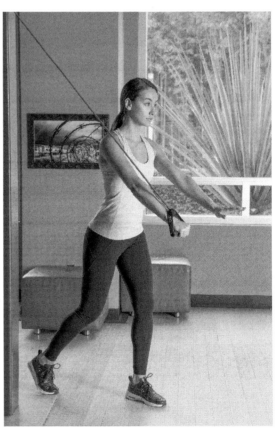

What it works: This pushing movement is designed to emphasize the chest, front delts and triceps along with Core Posture anti-rotation (don't twist).

How to do it: Secure the resistance band high in the door. Facing away from the resistance, place yourself in a stable split stance so that the opposite foot to the arm that you're pushing with is forward. Think about the dynamics of a two-arm regular chest press to guide you to the right position. Keep your body square and weight driven off the back leg from the ball of the foot. Start with both arms extended in front of you. Pretend your empty hand is pushing something to help stabilize that side and as you bring the loaded arm back, stretching your chest muscles, breathe in. Hold for a second and then breathe out as you drive the hand back to center line returning the chest to a shortened position.

Printed in Great Britain
by Amazon